THE PERSONALITY DISORDER TOOLBOX

The Challenge of the Hidden Agenda

Jeff Riggenbach, PhD
Award Winning Author of *The BPD Toolbox*

Copyright @2018 by Jeff Riggenbach

Cover: Matt Skar
Layout and Graphics: Dara Rogers

Book Versions:
Paperback ISBN: 9781730955655
eBook

All rights reserved

Printed in the United States of America

ENDORSEMENTS

Dr. Jeff Riggenbach delivers another must-have clinical manual with The Personality Disorders Toolbox! Filled with straight-forward exercises, handouts and worksheets as well as indispensable clinical guidance, this book streamlines the complex nature of treating personality disorders for therapists in the trenches. This book will be a "go to" resource for me and my staff when working with this population. Highly Recommended!"

— **Lane Pederson, PsyD, LP, DBPC**, author of the award-winning
The Expanded Dialectical Behavior Therapy Skills Training Manual, Second Edition

In "The Personality Disorder Toolbox," Dr. Riggenbach provides an invaluable resource for those of us who work with this difficult population. Anyone who works with personality disorders knows that these clients create confusion, drama, and upset, and Dr. Riggenbach's manual generously provides powerful counters to these difficulties with clear and specific concepts, forms, procedures, and guidelines. Any therapist working with personality disorders will find this manual to be tremendously helpful in planning, organizing, and facilitating treatment. We all owe Dr. Riggenbach a debt of gratitude for offering such a clear and helpful set of tools, I plan to keep his manual readily handy to use to offer more effective interventions for my clients.

— **Gregory W. Lester, Ph.D.**, author of
Diagnosis, Treatment, and Management of DSM 5 Personality Disorders

CONTENTS

About the Author 7

Introduction 9

Chapter 1
Personality Disorders 101 13

Chapter 2
Obsessive-Compulsive PD 29

Chapter 3
Avoidant PD 63

Chapter 4
Dependent PD 93

Chapter 5
Histrionic PD 127

Chapter 6
Antisocial PD 157

Chapter 7
Narcissistic PD 189

Chapter 8
Paranoid PD 221

Chapter 9
Borderline PD 255

Chapter 10
Schizoid and Schizotypal PDs 293

Conclusion 311

Bibliography 313

JEFF RIGGENBACH, PHD

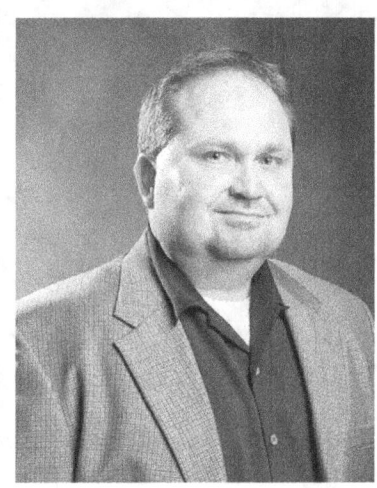

Jeff Riggenbach, PhD is a best selling author and an international speaker on the topic of personality disorders. He has spoken in all 50 United States and is on faculty of educational institutes in Canada, Australia, and South Africa. In total he has trained over 15,000 professionals world wide.

Dr. Riggenbach has devoted the past 20 years of his career to helping individuals with personality disorders, initially developing and directing treatment programs in psychiatric hospitals and outpatient clinics in which he participated in and oversaw the treatment of over 500 patients with Borderline PD. In recent years, he has shifted his focus to speaking, coaching, writing, and educating in an attempt to reduce the stigma associated with PDs and offer hope to those professionals and consumers who continue to believe the myth that recovery is not possible.

His most recent book, *The BPD Toolbox: A Practical, Evidence-Based Guide for Regulating Emotions* was extremely well received, and won silver publishing awards for best book in the areas of both psychology and self-help.

Jeff is a diplomat with the Academy of Cognitive Therapy, a Certified Cognitive Therapist, and currently serves as Director of the Personality Disorders Awareness Network. Contact him at bpdcoach@jeffriggenbach.com.

INTRODUCTION

Introduction

When I wrote my best selling *CBT Toolbox*, many people ask me "Can I use these tools with personality disorders?" I found this question difficult to answer. The correct answer was (and still is) "Yes, many of them, but you have to use them in different ways with different disorders and apply them differently to different people." While this is factually true, it is not a helpful answer. The obvious follow up questions were:

- Which tools?

- How do you apply them to different disorders?

- How to I know which tools are appropriate to use with which personality disordered population?

- What do you mean by applying them differently to specific people (many of whom may have the same disorder)?

These obviously aren't questions I could answer in a few minutes on break or at a book signing.

The majority of the personality disorder research and resources have been devoted to BPD and antisocial PD. Because Borderline PD is the most commonly seen disorder in the clinical setting, and the population I dealt with the most, I decided I would write a BPD toolbox. While I knew this book had a place, I was astonished to find out that it would become an award-winning book and be recognized as a Benjamin franklin silver winner in two categories. Most importantly, my heart has been warmed by the many letters I have received from people around the world who have benefitted from the tools in that book which were designed specifically for BPD.

However, I continued to get the same questions: "Can I use THESE tools with other personality disorders?"

Again, my answer would not satisfy most clinicians.

Although DSM 5 no longer utilizes a multiaxial diagnostic system, the significant differences that have always distinguished personality disorders from other disorders of clinical concern remain. Not only do personality disorders in general warrant their own designation, but each specific disorder has its own distinct cognitive, affective, and behavioral features which lend them to present in a variety of clinical and non-clinical settings. In addition to this, many individuals may not technically qualify for one specific disorder, but may have "traits" of many, which frequently seems to confuse clinicians regarding treatment approach.

So, in lieu of the above, I decided it was finally time to give each diagnosis the attention it deserves, so that each person with less "popular" personality disorders has a toolbox for their recovery as well. I mean, what if the medical community decided 'It's all just diabetes – there is no need to distinguish between type 1 and type 2?" If there were not a protocol for both types with interventions tailored specifically to respective types, many people would not be getting the treatment they need. As usual, individuals with personality disorders have remained underserved in a similar way. NO MORE! The Personality Disorder Toolbox will provide everything you need for treatment of ANY personality disorder. Not only will you have great new tools for treating Narcissists, Antisocials, and individuals with BPD, you will have a wide range of tools specifically tailored to EVERY personality disorder as well as tools for how to treat people with "traits" but no full-blown disorder. I hope you find this useful.

CHAPTER 1: PERSONALITY DISORDERS 101

What Makes a Personality Disorder?

Personality disorders (PDs) have been characterized by the Diagnostic and Statistical Manual of Mental Disorders (DSM) as "enduring patterns of inner experience and behavior that deviates markedly from the expectations of the individual's culture." These manifest in the following areas:

1. Cognition, i.e., ways of perceiving and interpreting self, others, and the world

2. Affectivity, relating to range and intensity of emotions

3. Interpersonal functioning, i.e., ability to get along with others

4. Impulse control

This all makes perfect sense on the surface level of course, because emotions (affect) are a product of thoughts (cognitions). Frequency of thoughts, content of thoughts, focus of thoughts, and meaning attached to thoughts are all a part of this. Emotions, or affect, influence our actions. When our cognitions interpret life events in extreme or distorted ways, it makes sense that we will experience intense emotions and act quickly (and often impulsively) in an attempt to diminish or alleviate them. Misperceiving the intent of others and acting in impulsive ways is clearly a good way to initiate or contribute to relational problems (interpersonal functioning).

So while this all makes sense on a surface level, the tools and exercises in this book will take you a little deeper.

By this explanation, everything starts with cognition. But where do our thoughts come from? They come from our beliefs.

While everyone has core beliefs, individuals with PDs have: 1) very specific combinations of beliefs; 2) much more *compelling* beliefs (that is, they hold them with greater degrees of conviction); and 3) beliefs which are more *pervasive* in nature, meaning they can be triggered in multiple areas of life, rather than in just one (such as a fear of public speaking).

Each chapter will address the specific belief combinations present in that particular disorder, as those are the driving forces responsible for problem thinking and behaviors. DSM lists behaviors, but people can act out the same behaviors with different "agendas." So it is the belief combinations that are really idiosyncratic and fuel specific symptom sets.

The purpose of this book is to offer you (whether you are an individual with a personality disorder or have a loved one with a personality disorder) a range of tools to help you identify and start to change those specific beliefs and behaviors. One consequence of having beliefs which are more compelling (or stronger) than the average person's: Those beliefs take much longer to change. For instance, the typical course of treatment for borderline personality disorder (BPD) is anywhere from one to four years.

Another consequence is that beliefs get *activated* with much more frequency. One of the more common colloquial expressions which many clients use to describe this experience is: "So-and-so really knows how to push my buttons." While we all have these "buttons" that get pushed, people with PDs feel emotions much more intensely than other people, which gives rise to impulsive behaviors that almost feel reflexive in nature to them. For many clients, it is helpful for them to have a mental image of a reflex (such as a physician's mallet tapping their knee or a similar "reflex reaction") to which they can relate. This provides a powerful way for people to gain awareness to these triggers which can easily influence their emotions and behavior; and thus their reactions to "pushed buttons" become less involuntary and they begin to feel empowered. Throughout the course of treatment, as these "buttons" become desensitized, so to speak, people are able to gain more self-control over their thoughts, feelings, and choices. Overall, the consequence of their beliefs being more compelling than other persons' is that not only are emotions more intense when those beliefs get activated, but they are activated much more frequently than others', usually in a wide variety of contexts in their lives.

In addition to having problems in the areas of cognition, affect, impulsivity, and relationships, it should be noted that unlike other disorders previously classified under "Axis I," PDs have been described as *ego-syntonic*, enduring, pervasive, and inflexible.

The term ego-syntonic was actually used in DSM-II, which came out in 1952. It was derived from the Freudian term "observing ego." Freud observed that individuals with PDs (though they were not called such at the time) lacked this observing ego—that is, they lacked the ability to objectively observe their own behavior. This is akin to what many would call having poor insight.

The term enduring refers to the fact that PDs don't "come and go" in a person's life in the same way that panic attacks or depressive episodes can. They endure over time.

Pervasive refers to the idea that has already been discussed—that these traits can show up in multiple areas of life.

Finally, PD behaviors are *inflexible*. This refers to the phenomenon that people with PDs have less ability to initiate different behaviors depending on what the situation calls for. For instance, people with histrionic personality disorder (HPD) can be flirtatious and attention-seeking whether or not it is appropriate for their current social setting. Flexibility, it should be noted, is one of the key factors that distinguishes someone who has a full-blown disorder from someone who may just have some of the traits or features of the condition but not be fully diagnosable.

Before giving you foundational information necessary for identifying and changing beliefs, cognitions, and behavior, it is necessary to address the issues of insight and flexibility.

. . .

I understand that some with personality disorders will not have the insight or flexibility to use the tools in the following chapters. Even at this point—prior to publication of this book—I have already received criticism for attempting to write it. But I would rather try and have it go over the head of some people than not follow through with this attempt and not help anyone. I'm reminded of the words of motivational speaker Les Brown: "Most people fail not because they aim too high and miss, but because they aim too low and hit." I want to help as many people as possible and don't want to be guilty of aiming too low.

I recall watching a training session by the legendary family systems therapist Bill O'Hanlon when I was in graduate school. He told a story about a time during one of his internships or similar kind of rotation in a psychiatric hospital as part of his training. He talked about sitting in on a treatment team meeting in which a certain telling event occurred. Anyone who has had the privilege of sitting through these meetings knows that they go a little something like this: A social worker reads down the census list reciting names of patients, and everyone on the treatment team in attendance will then give their update regarding each patient's treatment in the area of their particular discipline. These updates can vary greatly in length and detail, obviously, but each patient may get five minutes of discussion. In Bill's story, he describes how the social worker got to a particular patient's name, and the attending psychiatrist simply held two fingers up in the air in response; and upon this signal, everyone just started talking amongst themselves in a scattered way. Perplexed, he leaned over and asked the clinician next to him what in the world was happening. The person responded (I paraphrase here), "That means they have an Axis II condition—they have a personality disorder. Since there is nothing we can do for them anyway, we might as well just talk about whatever we want to."

I've probably butchered the story; that's what I get for telling someone else's personal anecdote. But the details are less important than the message. Twenty years later, having sitten through hundreds of these meetings myself, that story still sticks with me as a powerful portrayal of the longstanding attitude that has prevailed for so many years toward people with PDs.

Insight and flexibility are skills that can be developed with practice. Here are some tools that may help.

Developing Insight

All people have *blind spots:* parts of our personalities which others see in us but which we do not see in ourselves. Sometimes, it is helpful to have other people identify behaviors they see in us that they view as concerning, and then to be willing to take a hard look at how those behaviors might affect us in different areas.

Behaviors Others Have Expressed Concern Over	Areas These Behaviors Could Hurt Me
Behavior #1	Physically:
	Emotionally:
	Relationally:
	Spiritually:
	Financially:
	Legally:
Behavior #1	Physically:
	Emotionally:
	Relationally:
	Spiritually:
	Financially:
	Legally:

The following tool can help you develop some flexibility, as discussed above.

Developing Flexibility

All people have personality traits. Actually, all people have traits in each of the ten areas that the DSM would consider diagnosable. For instance, narcissism involves, in part, thinking highly of oneself. If you have acquired extensive training and/or knowledge in a particular field, then it is appropriate for you to see yourself as an expert in that field and feel confident in that view. However, narcissism becomes a problem when people view themselves as experts in areas that they actually are not, take on arrogant attitudes, and show low empathy for others.

Another diagnosis, HPD, is characterized by overly flirtatious or sexualized behavior, dramatic speech and/or behavior, and extremely shallow relationships. Having some histrionic traits may be helpful if one is single and trying to attract someone to date, or if they are a motivational speaker, or in theatre, and therefore being "dramatic" enhances their ability to entertain others. But these traits become disordered behavior if one is having sex with coworkers who are married to someone else; singing in the middle of a prayer at church; or engaging in loud and impulsive outbursts at a committee meeting, thus disrupting decision making.

There are eight other PDs we could go through in this way. But the point is that displaying traits associated with any of them isn't necessarily a bad thing. These traits can be helpful when harnessed appropriately. The reality is that life calls for us to act differently in different circumstances—in other words, what is appropriate in one context isn't necessarily appropriate in others. We have to be able to turn these traits "on" and "off," depending upon what is appropriate. We need to be able to behave differently when we are at a comedy club than we do when we are at a funeral. And the stronger a person exhibits these traits, the more difficult navigating these behaviors can be for them.

Use the following tool to help you identify traits that you have, as well as areas that these traits could be HELPFUL to you and areas they could be HURTFUL to you.

Personality Flexibility Tool

A Few Examples:

Trait	Helpful to Me	Hurtful to Me
Critical Mind	Good at analyzing what's wrong with cars brought into the shop.	Overly critical of my wife and kids at home.
Emotional Intensity	Passionate in relationships. When things are good, they are really good.	Too sensitive. I get my feelings hurt and become angry with people too easily.

Trait	Helpful to Me	Hurtful to Me

- One change I will make this week to minimize the way my traits have been hurting me is _____
_____
_____

- One change I will make this week to maximize the way my traits have been helping me is _____
_____
_____

Treatment That Has Failed

Once some insight has been developed and at least minimal motivation exists, it is time for treatment. However, many people believe PDs are untreatable. Let's take a moment to look at why that is.

Firstly, anyone who still believes this does not follow current research. The sad reality is that many people don't keep up with scientific advancement or simply make global assumptions based on their experiences.

Secondly, and to give the naysayers a little benefit of the doubt, in the past it was true that treatments were NOT effective. When these diagnoses were first starting to be understood, psychoanalysts ruled the psychological world. And while their work provided much needed early understanding, it offered little to nothing in the way of practical help. Since early psychoanalysis could not treat PDs, and psychoanalytic treatments were just about all we had in the 1960s, it is understandable that many arrived at this belief. An unhelpful byproduct of the times was that the majority of professionals teaching in university settings were psychoanalytically trained; and thus many students were taught that "nothing works" in graduate school.

Unfortunately, things seem to change slowly in this field. It amazes me how many graduate programs still seem to have that one course in psychopathology that contains only one segment in it on PDs, and as a result many mental health professionals are inadequately trained to treat PDs. In fact, many master's degree programs offer excellent training for the treatment of depression, anxiety, and other general disorders of clinical concern; but it is problematic that many psychologists and therapists graduate to use those same techniques to treat PDs. You don't treat a bone fracture with a multivitamin prescription. So while the strategies which most professionals in the mental health field know can help in general ways, they aren't nearly specific enough to treat PDs.

To quote Mark Twain: "If all you have is a hammer, everything looks like a nail." This phenomenon seems to have played a significant role in past treatment failure.

Treatment That Succeeds

There are likely many other contributing factors to why treatment has historically failed. But enough with the negativity. Let's get to treatment that works! A number of therapies have now been shown to be evidence based: namely, Dialectical Behavior Therapy (DBT), Cognitive Behavior Therapy (CBT), Schema-focused Therapy (SFT), and Mentalization-based Treatment (MBT). This workbook will draw largely from these modalities.

Since DSM 5 defines personality disorders in terms of disturbance in cognition, affect, interpersonal function, and impulsivity, this book will organize its tools accordingly.

As mentioned above, we have each gone through unique experiences in life that shape how we view things. These experiences help create what are often called our core beliefs or schemas. Although technically, these two terms don't share exactly the same meaning, this workbook uses the terms interchangeably.

Our definition for both is "a mental filter that guides how people interpret events." Judith Beck, President of the Beck Institute for Cognitive Behavior Therapy, created a visual of a schema that looks like this:

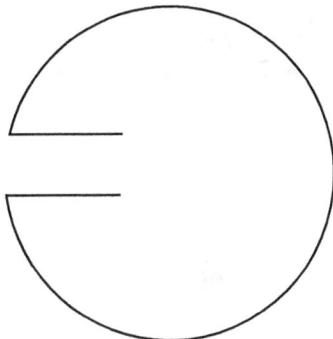

© J. Beck, 2005. Adapted from Cognitive Therapy for Challenging Problems and used with permission. www.beckinstitute.org

It looks a little like a backwards Pac-man. Take for example a woman who has a belief that "others won't approve of me." Pretend she overhears one of the mums at her daughter's day care say "I wish the girls were more talkative." How might you guess she will interpret that? It would likely look something like this:

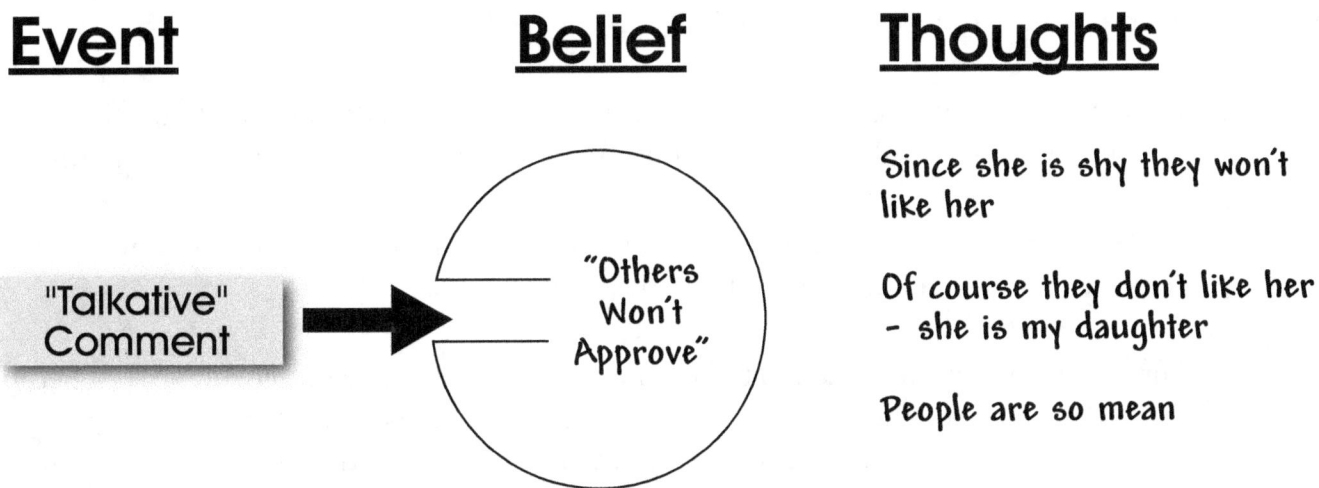

Now, assume that 4 other mums praised her daughter saying they thought she was sweet and she hoped that they could be friends. How might her filter/belief interpret those statements?

Chapter 1: Personality Disorders 101

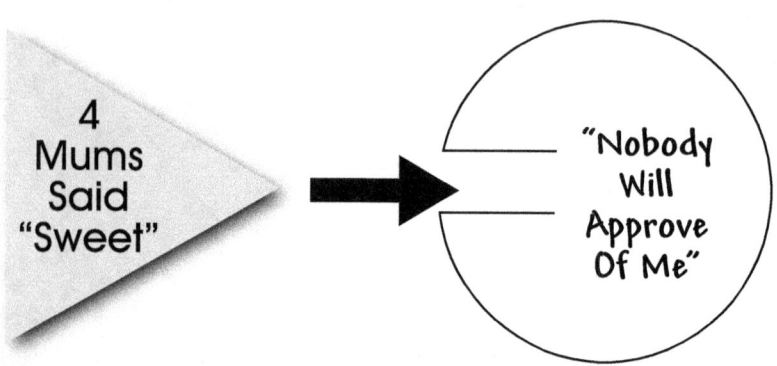

Can you see the role of the filter here? Any information that is consistent with the belief (represented by rectangles) would "fit" the opening of the figure, whereby allowing it to "go in" straight to the belief. These events or comments produce intense feelings.

Any information that is inconsistence with the belief (represented by triangles) would not "fit." If they tried to "enter the figures" they would hit and "bounce off" producing a distorted interpretation.

In the top example, the woman took a comment that was not even directed at her daughter and made it mean (i.e., perceived it as) something critical and disapproving.

The second comment was clearly intended to be personal and was in fact favorable for her, but because it didn't "fit" her belief, she discounted it and was not able to hear it as it was intended. So it is easy to see how those attempting to communicate with individuals often say things like "I can't win." As will be discussed later in the book, although this is often perceived as manipulation or "not trying," this response is genuinely how people with PDs process information. So this is really how they think and feel.

A big part of treatment, then, is directed at lessening the strength of distorted filters such as this. Doing so reduces misperceptions and misinterpretations and any resulting disagreements.

Another long term goal, then, is to not only chisel away at the unhealthy belief, but also to work at constructing and enlarging an alternate belief.

A visual for an alternate adaptive belief might look like the one on the next page.

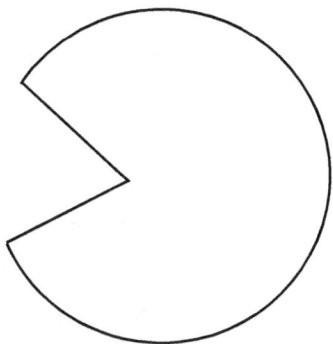

This is a structure that one of those triangles could fit into. Now consider how the same two events (comments in this case) might have been received differently if this young lady had an alternate belief.

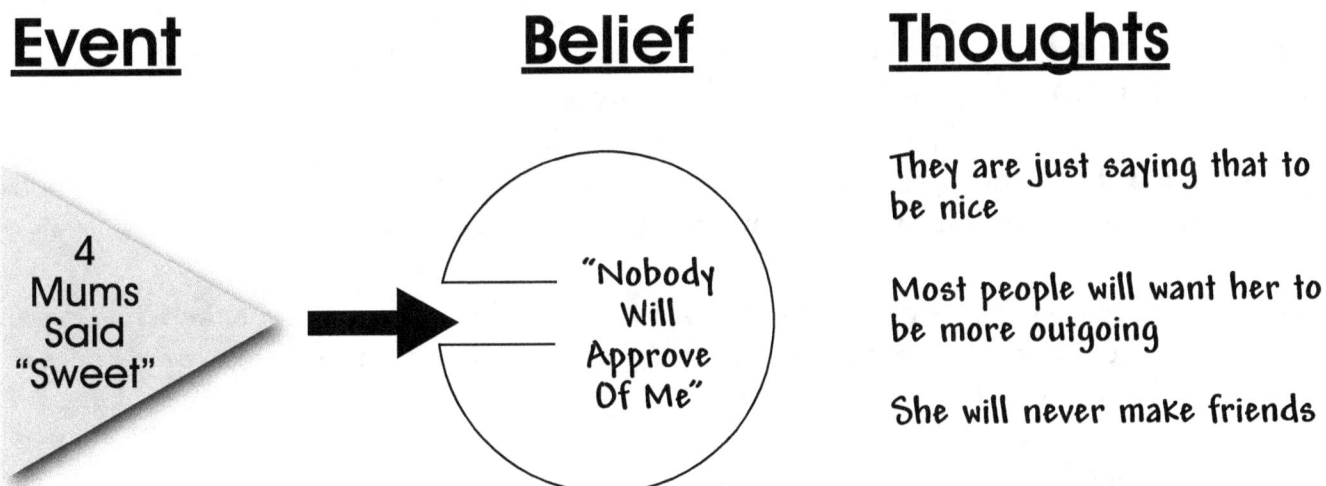

In this case, a neutral statement could be interpreted in a more open, flexible way, thereby contributing less intense negative or perhaps even hopeful emotions.

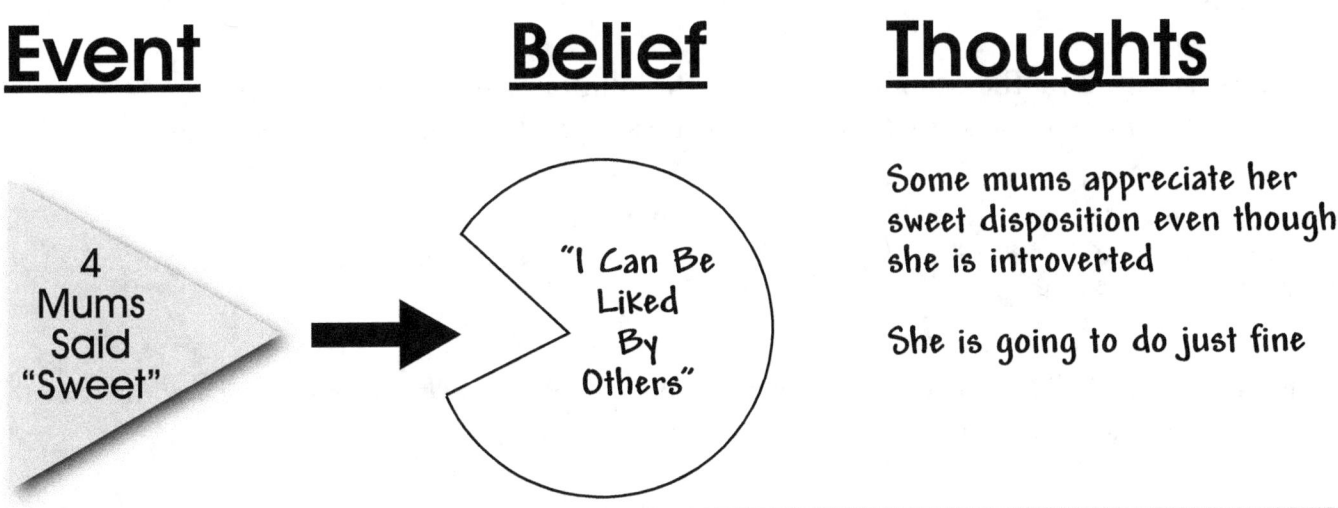

And, in the case where the comment was clearly meant to be positive, she could receive the statement in the manner that it was intended, and experience positive emotions.

So, now that you have a basic understanding of the roles which beliefs play in information processing, review the following list of Jeff Young's schemas to get an idea of the content present in each. These will play a central role in the tools introduced in each chapter in this book.

Failure: The belief that one isn't good enough, can't do anything right, or is a loser.

Approval-Seeking Mindset/Unlovability or Unlikability: The belief that one is not likable or lovable, that nobody cares about one, and that one can't make or keep friends or romantic relationships; and one is perturbed (as opposed to unfazed) by these thoughts. This is the belief that comes into play for "people-pleasers."

Helplessness: The belief that one can't cope, either with a particular situation or with life in general. This core belief leads to feelings of inadequacy and anxiety.

Worthlessness/Defectiveness: The belief that one has no value, is unworthy, or is "damaged goods." For some people, these three qualities feel similar, and for others, they are different.

Abandonment: The belief that significant others in one's life will leave or won't be there for one, and that one will not be able to tolerate being alone. People with this belief may go to extreme measures to keep from being alone.

Mistrust: The belief that others are untrustworthy, out to get one, or otherwise not looking out for one's best interest. This is a core belief that leads people to become overly suspicious or outright paranoid.

Vulnerability: There are different versions of this belief, as it can show up in different areas of life, but in general, this is the belief that one is unsafe and in some way (relationally, medically, financially, etc.) overly susceptible to being hurt. People with this belief interpret events in life as more threatening than they really are.

Emotional Inhibition: The belief that one must inhibit one's emotions—not speak up or not share thoughts or feelings—because to do so would be unacceptable or harmful in some way.

Emotional Deprivation: The belief that one will not get emotional needs met, so one often doesn't try. Some people with this belief will say, "I don't have needs;" "Your needs are more important than mine;" or "It's weak to have needs."

Subjugation: This belief is related to control. Some people believe they must turn control of their lives over to others, while others make efforts not to be controlled or controlling. If you have "control issues," this belief is involved.

Entitlement: The belief that one is special or in some way better or more deserving than others. Often, this belief serves to cover up an underlying insecurity (defectiveness, emotional deprivation, etc.): People who feel insecure but do not want to be seen as fragile may adopt a "tough guy/girl" facade. However, some were raised from childhood with no limits and really do view themselves as better than others.

Punishment: The belief that one deserves to be punished. Punishment can be directed toward self or others. Our society has become quite litigious due to this belief. There are some psychiatric patients and inmates who just can't wait to file a grievance. Sadistic, masochistic, and self-harming behaviors may also be products of this belief.

Insufficient Self-Control: The belief that produces the cognition, "I have to have it now." These people believe that they have no self-control and no ability to restrain themselves or to delay gratification in the "heat of the moment." Impulsive substance abuse, sexual promiscuity, binge eating, temper tantrums, and shopping sprees may be products of this belief.

These core beliefs produce certain cognitive distortions, or misperceptions, to which diagnostic criteria refer; that is they guide people's thoughts about situations in unhelpful, extreme or inaccurate ways. Although, Dr. Beck identified the existence of these in the 1960s in some of his initial work with depressed patients, I want to point out that Dr. David Burns wrote one of the best self-help books in 1980 explaining and describing these in lay terms. All these years later, and even with all of the new areas of emphasis in the broader arena of cognitive psychology, these remain a staple of our programs and in my opinion are still one of the most practical ways to help clients identify and work to change their lives in fundamental ways.

Specific distortions will be referenced in each chapter throughout the book as they pertain to the PD being addressed. Having an understanding of these is vital to your ability to link thought processes to certain behaviors and thus really to comprehend the rest of this book.

Cognitive Distortions

What follows are ten misperceptions, or cognitive distortions, that form the basis for your emotional difficulties (adapted from Burns, 1990).

1. Rationalization. In an attempt to protect yourself from hurt feelings, you create excuses for events in life that don't go your way or for poor choices you make. We might call these permission-giving statements that give ourselves or someone else permission to do something that is in some way unhealthy.

2. Overgeneralization. You categorize different people, places, and entities based on your own experiences with each particular thing. For example, if you have been treated poorly by men in the past, "all men are mean;" or if your first wife cheated on you, "all women are unfaithful." By overgeneralizing, you miss out on experiences that don't fit your particular stereotype. This is the distortion on which all of those "-isms" (e.g., racism, sexism) are based.

3. All-or-nothing thinking. This refers to a tendency to see things in black-and-white categories with no consideration for gray areas. You see yourself, others, and often the whole world in only positive or negative extremes rather than considering that each may instead have both positive and negative aspects. For example, if your performance falls short of perfect, you see yourself as a total failure. If you catch yourself using extreme language ("best ever," "worst," "love," "hate," "always," "never"), it is a red flag that you may be engaging in all-or-nothing thinking. This extreme thinking leads to intense feelings and an inability to see a "middle ground" perspective or feel proportionate moods.

4. Discounting the positive. You reject positive experiences by insisting that they "don't count" for some reason or another. In this way, you can maintain a negative belief that is contradicted by your everyday experiences. The terms mental filter and selective abstraction basically describe the same process.

5. Fortune telling. You anticipate that things will turn out badly and feel convinced that your prediction is already an established fact based on your experiences from the past. Predicting a negative outcome before any outcome occurs leads to anxiety and other negative emotions. A lot of people call this process the "what-ifs."

6. Mind reading. Rather than predicting future events, engaging in this distortion involves predicting that you know what someone else is thinking when in reality you don't. This distortion commonly occurs in communication problems between romantic partners.

7. "Should" statements. You place false or unrealistic expectations on yourself or others, thereby setting yourself up to feel angry, guilty, or disappointed. Words and phrases such as ought to, must, has to, needs to, and supposed to are indicative of "should" thinking.

8. Emotional reasoning. You assume that your negative feelings reflect the way things really are. For example: "I feel it, therefore it must be true."

9. Magnification. You exaggerate the importance of things, blowing them way out of proportion. Often, this takes the form of fortune telling and/or mind reading to an extreme. This way of thinking may also be referred to as catastrophizing or awfulizing.

10. Personalization. You see yourself as the cause of some external negative event for which, in fact, you were not primarily responsible. You make something about you that is not about you and get your feelings hurt.

So the readers' digest version is this: We have all developed beliefs as a result of our life experiences and the meaning that we have attributed to those experiences. (Biology plays a role here as well.) Beliefs get activated (or "buttons get pushed") by various life events or physiological sensations or symptoms. As we get triggered, the beliefs filter our thinking in certain ways, which are often biased or distorted. Distorted thinking often leads to uncomfortable emotions, which often drive our choices, which in turn produce consequences in our lives. A simplified version of the broader model of cognitive-behavioral based approaches (which include DBT and SFT) for treatment and coaching provides a helpful visual for a lot of people.

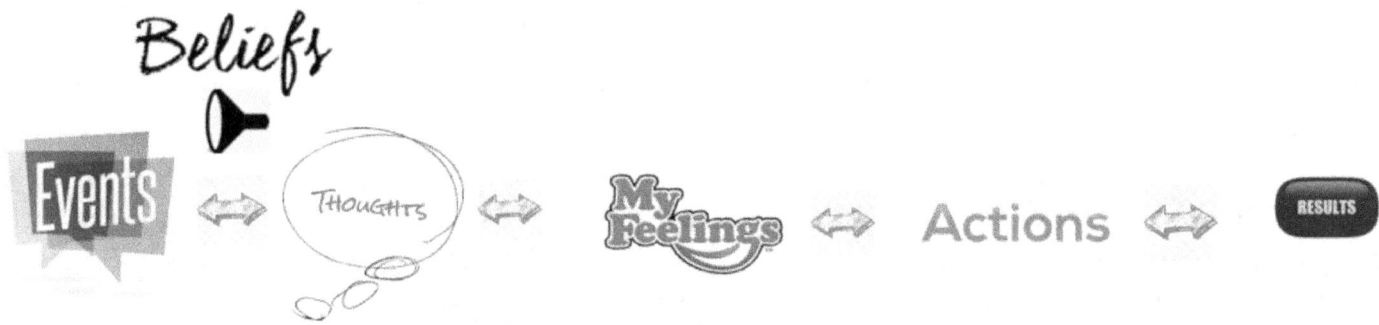

People with PDs have stronger unhealthy beliefs and have more "buttons" than those without PDs, and those unhealthy beliefs are often much more deeply ingrained. Thus thoughts are more extreme, emotions more intense, and behaviors more erratic, impulsive, and oftentimes self-destructive.

This book will help you identify what belief constellations, thought processes, and emotional responses are common in each of the disorders that are producing the behaviors that do so much damage to the individual suffering from the PD as well as others in their lives. And, then, most importantly, it will give you specific and practical tools to add to your therapeutic toolbox that will equip you or your clients on the journey toward recovery!

What Are the Personality Disorders?

General characteristics of PDs have been described above. Here are brief explanations of the specific disorders. More detail will be offered in their respective chapters.

Obsessive-Compulsive Personality Disorder – This is the extreme perfectionist. They have very rigid ideas about what is "right" in the world and expect others to adhere to their expectations.

Avoidant Personality Disorder – People with avoidant tendencies have an excessive fear of being judged. For this reason, they are unusually reluctant to enter relationships or even take jobs that require interaction with people.

Dependent Personality Disorder – This person has an excessive fear of being alone, which often manifests in "needy" behaviors in relationships. This also can include difficulty taking responsibility in basic areas of life.

Histrionic Personality Disorder – This person needs to be the life of the party. They will exhibit flirtatious, sexually provocative, and other attention-seeking behavior. They can also have shallow mood swings.

Antisocial Personality Disorder – This person has a disregard for rules, expectations, and people. Many with moderate to severe versions of this have run-ins with the law and spend some time incarcerated.

Narcissistic Personality Disorder – This person lacks empathy, displays an exaggerated sense of self-importance, and often comes across as a bully.

Borderline Personality Disorder – This is the most "popular" of the PDs and is seen most often in mental health clinics and psychiatric hospitals. People with BPD struggle with abandonment issues, deregulated emotions, and impulsive/destructive behaviors, amongst other things.

Paranoid Personality Disorder – This person struggles with pervasive mistrust of other people, suspiciousness regarding being exploited, and deep-seated anger with excessive grudge holding.

Schizoid Personality Disorder – This person is detached and indifferent. They prefer time alone rather than with people and don't really care what anyone else thinks.

Schizotypal Personality Disorder – The person with this disorder has unusual beliefs, strange behavior, and can be socially awkward. This PD has some association with schizophrenia.

CHAPTER 2: THE OBSESSIVE COMPULSIVE PERSONALITY DISORDER

The Obsessive Compulsive Personality Disorder

Hidden agenda: To follow the rules

Prevalence rates: Approximately 2-8% of the general population

Gender distribution: More commonly diagnosed in men than women

Cognitive profile:

- "I must be responsible," "I must be orderly"

- "Others are irresponsible," "Others are messy," "Others should do better"

- "The rules must be followed," "Details are important"

Common schemas: Failure, unrelenting standards, emotional inhibition, negativity

Common cognitive distortions:

- "Should" statements (towards self, others, and world)

- Discounting the positive

Overdeveloped traits: Control, responsibility

Underdeveloped traits: Spontaneity, playfulness

Whom they date/marry: Histrionics; others who express emotionality and "have fun"

Where they work: Accountants, Quality control, Computer systems analysts and other IT positions

Other Random Nuggets:

- Some view as a marker of severity for obsessive compulsive disorder (OCD)

- Most common at the trait level in the general population

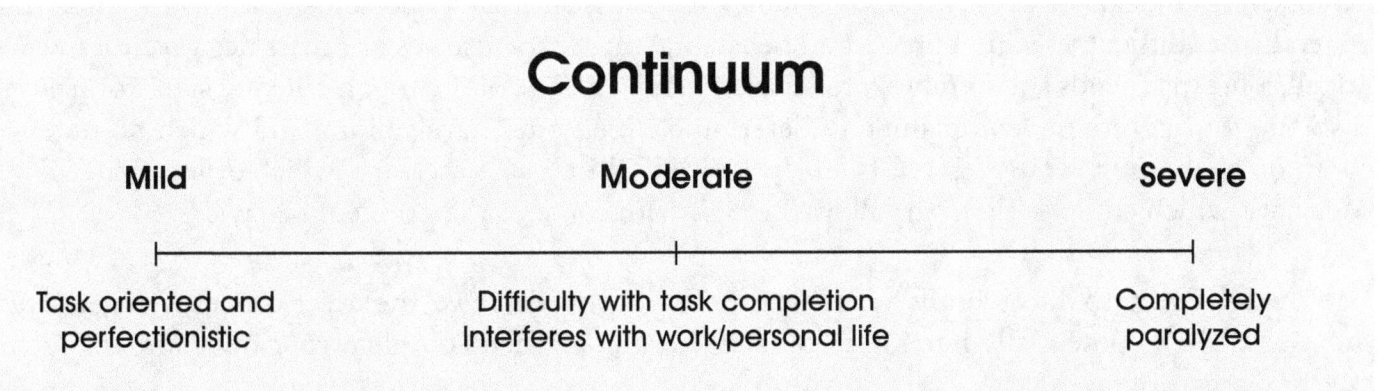

Tool #1: Trait Checklist

Individuals that suffer from the characteristics of obsessive-compulsive personality disorder (OCPD) have a number of commonalities. Whether you or a loved one has this full blown condition, or some of the traits of it, survey the following checklist. The more of these you checkmark, the more likely it is this pattern of behavior is causing some problems occupationally, relationally, or socially.

- ❑ Inability to delegate
- ❑ Rigid
- ❑ Easily annoyed
- ❑ Low-level anger
- ❑ Preoccupied with details
- ❑ Stingy with money
- ❑ Has a "right" and "wrong" way of doing things that has nothing to do with true morality

- ❑ Stubborn
- ❑ Extremely dedicated to work
- ❑ Perfectionism that interferes with task completion
- ❑ Relationships that take on a serious quality
- ❑ Lack spontaneity
- ❑ Control issues in relationships
- ❑ Play time is work time

Chapter 2: The Obsessive Compulsive Personality Disorder

Tool #2: Expressions of Concern

All people have what are often called "blind spots": qualities we don't see in ourselves as well as others see in us. Because of the ego-syntonic nature of PDs, this phenomenon is particularly challenging for these people. What this means practically is that things that pose problems for friends and family members are often not are considered as problematic by the individual with the condition. Concerns expressed friends and family may have validity to them, but due to poor insight, the PD individual generally has difficulty seeing how certain behaviors impact themselves or others negatively. However, not all concerns friends and family express have validity. So, one of the tough but vital steps for recovery is sorting through these "complaints" to determine which ones have validity and which do not. One common challenge people with OCPD have is seeing things as "necessary" which others don't view as necessary, which compels them to follow through with some of the problem behaviors.

Use the following tool to identify *who* has expressed concern, *what* the exact concerns are, and *why* they see them as potentially hurtful. Look at the example, then complete your own and answer the questions that follow.

Example:

Person Expressing Concern	Action Causing Concern	Reason for Concern
1. Boss	1. Difficulty accomplishing work	1. Job at risk
2. Wife	2. Working long hours	2. Marital problems
3. Children	3. Not enough "dad time"	3. Miss their dad
4. Mother	4. Look stressed these days	4. Possible health effects
5. Friend Dave	5. Never make it to guys' night anymore"	5. Not sure he is "ok"

Questions:

- Who are three people I trust to "shoot straight" with me, by whom I can run these concerns to get their opinion?

    1. Friend Dave

    2. Mom

    3. High school coach

- With which concerns can I at least see where the "complainer" is coming from?

    Don't want to lose my job

- I am willing to take the following steps to change one of the concerns:

    1. Go to therapy

    2. Monitor my work hours closer

    3. Schedule two "fun hours" per week (even if it feels like I am behind)

My Expressions of Concern

Person Expressing Concern	Action Causing Concern	Reason for Concern
1.	1.	1.
2.	2.	2.
3.	3.	3.
4.	4.	4.
5.	5.	5.

Questions:

- Who are three people I trust to "shoot straight" with me, by whom I can run these concerns by to get their opinion?

    1. _____

    2. _____

    3. _____

- Which concerns can I at least see where the "complainer" is coming from?

_____

_____

Chapter 2: The Obsessive Compulsive Personality Disorder

- I am willing to take the following steps to change one of the concerns

    1. _____

    2. _____

    3. _____

Tool #3: Pros and Cons

This tool helps you evaluate the potential pros and cons of your perfectionism behaviors. It is called a *four box pros and cons*. Sometimes it can be beneficial to look at not only the advantages and disadvantages of maintaining certain behaviors but also the advantages and disadvantages of changing them. After listing the pros and cons of each, it can be even more helpful to rate, on a scale of 0-10, how important each item is. Consider the example that is provided. Then complete one on your own!

Example: Pros and Cons of Perfectionistic Behavior

Pros of Remaining Perfectionistic	Pros of Slight Lowering of Standards
Get it right (9)	Get projects done sooner (5)
Cover all the details (9)	Get home sooner (6)
Don't have to worry something is missing (8)	Minimize overtime (7)
	More time with kids (7)
	Happier wife (10)
	Boss happier with me (10)
Cons of Remaining Perfectionistic	**Cons of Slight Lowering of Standards**
Could lose my job (10)	Feels "Sloppy" (7)
Could lose my marriage (10)	
May upset friends on committee (6)	
Come across as critical of others when I don't mean to be (6)	
Have lost friends (6)	

Results:

__26__ Reasons to remain perfectionistic

__38__ Reasons to not

__45__ Reasons to lower standards

__7__ Reasons to not lower standards

My Pros and Cons of Perfectionistic Behavior

Pros of Remaining Perfectionistic	Pros of Slight Lowering of Standards
Cons of Remaining Perfectionistic	**Cons of Slight Lowering of Standards**

Results:

_____ Reasons to remain perfectionistic

_____ Reasons to Lower Standards

_____ Reasons to lower standards

_____ Reasons to Lower Standards

My Conclusions _____
_____
_____
_____

My Commitment(s) _____
_____
_____
_____
_____

Tool #4: Identify Behavioral Targets

Perfectionism manifests differently in different people. Some behaviors include: regularly reorganizing house or office, overanalyzing when making decisions, taking longer than desired to complete tasks, working overtime, coming home late, difficulty completing projects around the house, garage, or yard, becoming irritable and snapping at other people, "redoing" work or projects others have done because they did not quite do it correctly, difficulty approximating or giving estimates, becoming critical of others, and countless more.

Use this tool to identify some of your perfectionistic behaviors that you or others have noticed. Feel free to use any of the above behaviors that fit, or list some of your own.

- Behaviors related to my perfectionism traits that I or someone else identified which I am willing to target to improve my situation

    1. _____
    2. _____
    3. _____
    4. _____
    5. _____

Tool #5: Intimacy Circles

Intimacy is a scary word for a lot of people. If the sound of it makes you cringe, this exercise is definitely for you—and even if it doesn't, this exercise likely will still benefit you. It will benefit almost everyone in some way. Why? Because almost everyone could benefit from improving at least one interpersonal relationship in their life. Some people's lives could be enriched with more friends. Others need to learn to set boundaries with someone in their life. A lot of people have "trust issues." Yet others would be happier in life if they learned to pick healthier people to date or form friendships with; toxic people have a way of draining people of their energy and joy. A certain percentage of the population would be much less prone to mood swings if they could be okay alone. Some would find more fulfillment in life if they could share more with people in their lives; others would not be hurt as often if they learned to share less with those in their life. A lot of people walk around with their "walls" up. Some have difficulty expressing feelings. Some have been accused of being too "needy." Others have difficulty asking for help.

You may have heard intimacy defined as "Into-Me-See"——the degree to which we let people see into us, and vice versa. A lot of my clients have found this "play on words" to be a helpful way to remember its definition and connotations.

Use the following tool to evaluate the relationships in your life. Use the percentage signs to help you decide which people to put in which circles. No other person goes in the ME circle (though some people choose to put God here). This is for you alone. People who belong in circle #1 are those with whom you would feel comfortable sharing ANY problem in life, no matter how personal (a sexual problem, something related to an abusive situation, a salary issue, etc.). People in circle #2 are those in your life with whom there may be a personal issue or two (like the ones mentioned above) that you would not share, but you would be comfortable sharing ALMOST anything (roughly 75%) about your life. People in circle #3 may get about half of your personal stuff, but the other half you probably would not trust them with. People in circle #4 would be your very casual relationships. Maybe they know whether you are married or where you work or something of that nature, but you don't share very much with them (roughly 25%). And people in circle #5 get nothing. For some people, these are individuals

whom they have just met, so they could be candidates to move closer in as they get to know them. Or, these are people who at one point in life were closer in, but they have done something to violate trust, so they have had to be moved out one or more rings.

Perfectionistic individuals value task completion over relationships, but that does not mean they aren't interested in relationships. Others may find them frustrating to be in relationships with due to 1) high standards for themselves that influence them away from relational activities, and 2) high standards for others that can produce annoyance in the person with OCPD traits, as well as a feeling of often being criticized by the people they are in relationships with. If this is you, keep in mind that even though you likely view your standards as "the correct ones," others view them as unnecessary. Practice empathy and try to consider how these standards might affect your relationships.

Keep these ideas in mind as you consider who truly belongs where as you complete your circles. Your first task is to think about all the people in your life and where they go in your circles. Then consider the questions that follow to get you started making healthy changes to your relationships. Work with your therapist or other helping professional if you need ongoing guidance or accountability.

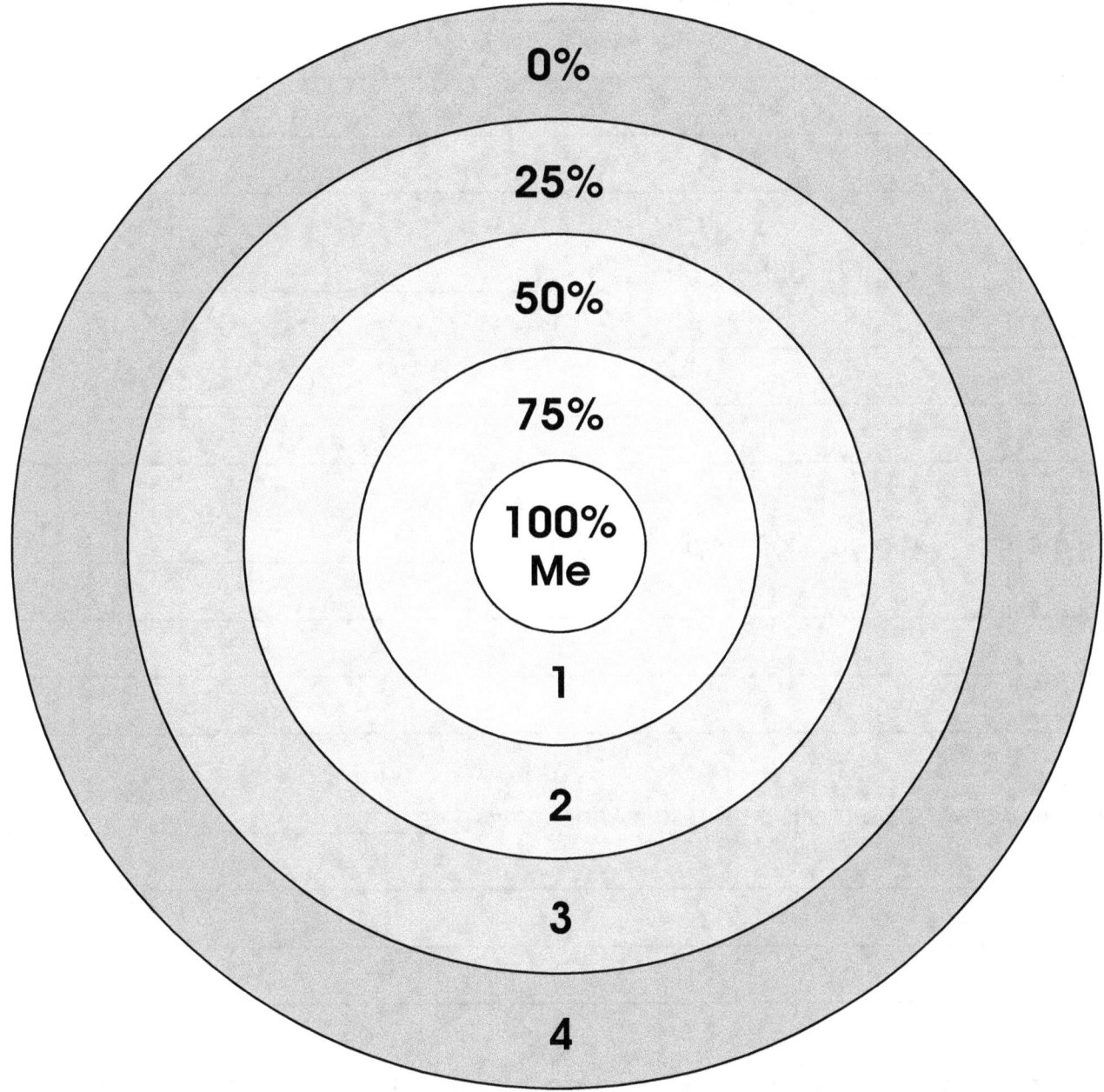

Intimacy Circles Follow-Up Starter Questions

- General observations about my circles _____
_____
_____
_____

- What I like most about my circles _____
_____
_____
_____

- What I like least about my circles _____
_____
_____
_____

- The most problematic people in my life _____
_____
_____
_____

- They are problematic in the following ways _____
_____
_____
_____

- People in my life whose opinions I actually care about and on a scale of 0-10 how much I care what they think _____
_____
_____
_____

- People in my life whose opinions I don't care about _____
_____
_____

- People in my life whom I have hurt/violated/taken advantage of _____
  _____
  _____
  _____

- People in my life who have moved themselves out in my circles due to my behavior _____
  _____
  _____
  _____

- I could improve my circles if I were willing to keep the following rules (which I have not previously been willing to keep) _____
  _____
  _____
  _____

- One step I will take TODAY to improve my relationship circles _____
  _____
  _____
  _____

Tool #6: Identify and Restructure Automatic Thoughts

A staple component of treatment for any psychological condition is recognizing the thought processes that are driving the problem behaviors and maintaining the symptoms. In colloquial language, you may hear this referred to as "self-talk." To speak in the terms of the Mark Twain quote in the introduction ("If all you have is a hammer, everything looks like a nail"): This is the "hammer." While treatment of personality disorders requires more tools than just a hammer, the hammer is still a useful tool to have in your toolbox.

Some people develop an awareness of their thoughts and get better at noticing them, but do nothing to change them. For example, if we recognize that we are overweight, but do nothing to change our diets

or exercise levels, we will stay overweight. In the same way, if we recognize thoughts that are driving problem behavior but do nothing to change them, our symptoms are likely to remain.

So, one cognitive tool you can use is what is called challenging distorted thoughts when you recognize them. Refer to the beginning of this chapter for some distorted thoughts common in obsessive compulsive personality disorder. *"Challenging,"* in this case, basically means "arguing" with the specific content of the thoughts. There are a number of techniques that can be used for doing this, including looking at evidence, seeking input from others, researching the facts, considering past or possible future results, or good old-fashioned logic, just to name a few.

The following tool asks you to identify specific obsessive compulsive thoughts that enter your mind, challenge them in some way, and if you want to, rate your challenge on a scale of 0-10, indicating how meaningful the challenge is. Take a look at the example, and then do one on your own. This may be a tool that you will benefit from using on an ongoing basis.

Example: Thought Log

Distorted Thought	Rational Responses
I have to complete this project before I go home. I must do it perfectly. If it is not of the highest quality, it isn't good enough.	My deadline isn't tonight I promised my wife I would be home by six tonight. I know she made plans for once and it is a special occasion.
I need to start over. It has to be just right.	High quality is important, but my 70% is better than other people's 100%. My supervisor has already signed off on this part of the project, and he has made it clear he doesn't want to pay me any more overtime this period. I don't need to go back and redo it. Go home and have a nice evening with my wife

Thought Log

Distorted Thought	Rational Responses

Tool #7: Historical Experiences Worksheet

As with most, if not all, personality disorders, there are multiple pathways to OCPD. Although it is known that this PD has at least a moderate genetic component, many people with these traits do have some commonalities in their backgrounds of experience. Peruse the following historical experiences worksheet and put an "X" beside factors that were a part of your experiences from a young age.

- ❏ Routine was emphasized from a young age
- ❏ Parents were rigid
- ❏ Parents were controlling
- ❏ Parents emphasized performance
- ❏ Felt coerced to follow rules from a young age
- ❏ Perfectionism trait in primary caretaker(s) from a young age
- ❏ Honest mistakes were looked down upon or punished
- ❏ Caretaker(s) demonstrated little warmth or emotional support from a young age
- ❏ Was taught to control emotions or that it was not okay to express feelings from a young age

- Describe how the experiences checked above apply specifically to you and the impact you believe they continue to have in your life today

_____
_____
_____
_____
_____
_____
_____
_____
_____
_____

Tool #8: Belief Identification

As has been discussed, all behaviors are a product of beliefs. Beliefs drive behavior. Due to the compelling nature of beliefs in individuals with PDs, these deeper-level beliefs often have to be modified to help create lasting change. As noted at the beginning of this chapter, common beliefs in people with OCPD include failure, unrelenting standards, emotional inhibition, and negativity. Review their definitions if you don't have them fresh in your mind. Get with your therapist. Include friends and family who are willing to give you feedback. Identify one or two beliefs that you believe drive your target behaviors to work on in treatment. Write them inside Judy Beck's "Pac-Man" visual aid (which was explained in the introduction).

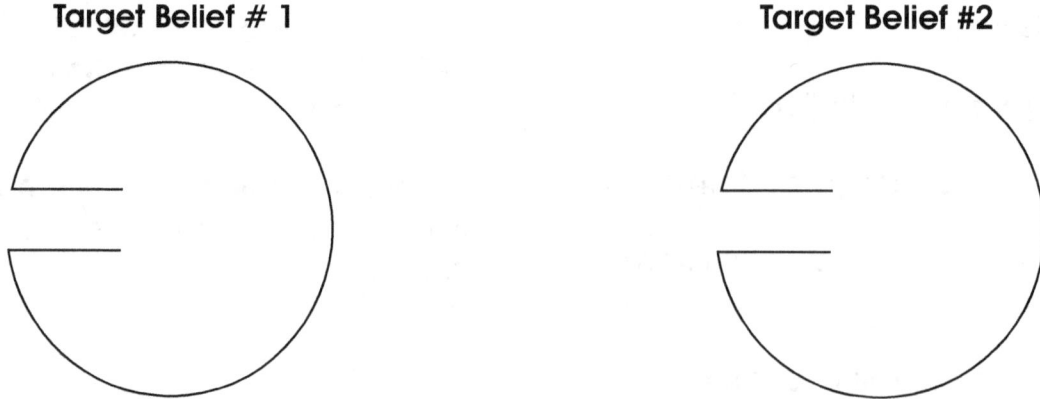

Beliefs always come in pairs. For every maladaptive (or unhealthy) belief we have, we also possess an alternate, adaptive (or healthy) belief. For instance, even though an individual may have the belief, "I am a failure," they also have the belief, however faint, "I can succeed." Every person that has a belief that they are worthless also has an opposite belief that they can have some value.

I have given you the "pushing buttons" language, the "Pac-Man" visual, and the "filters" imagery. Here is another representation which I hope helps illustrate the point: We could think of beliefs as lenses. For people who wear glasses, this visual probably comes fairly intuitively. Healthier individuals are able to engage in more balanced information processing. Figuratively speaking they are able to see out of both the left and the right "lenses" equally. This is the goal of belief modification work: balanced information processing. In other words, to be able to see both sides objectively and to be able to recognize when they fail or make mistakes, so they can learn from them; and also to be able to acknowledge when they succeed and be able to take a compliment. Although nobody is perfect and everyone has their biases, healthier people's lenses are closer to the 50/50 range (50% failure/50% success). Before treatment, people with PDs, due to their more compelling beliefs, often start with numbers such as 99%/1%. *Intentional and sustained effort* is required to create a healthier belief balance.

So, now that you have identified your unhealthy beliefs driving your target behaviors, identify, in your own words, what you would call the opposite, healthy belief. Write it in the opposite belief structure that the "triangle" could fit into.

After you have identified your one to two healthy and unhealthy beliefs, ask your self: What percentage of the time do I believe the unhealthy belief? What percentage of the time do I believe the healthy belief? Write your numbers in the line next to each belief. (they should total 100%). Then you are ready to move on to Tool #9!

See the example first, and then do one on your own!

Example: Belief Identification

Target Belief #1	Healthy Belief #1
"Unrelenting Standards"	"Doesn't Have to be Perfect/exact"
90% Strength	10% Strength
Target Belief #2	**Healthy Belief #2**
"Critical"	"Can Give Some Grace"
80% Strength	20% Strength

My Beliefs

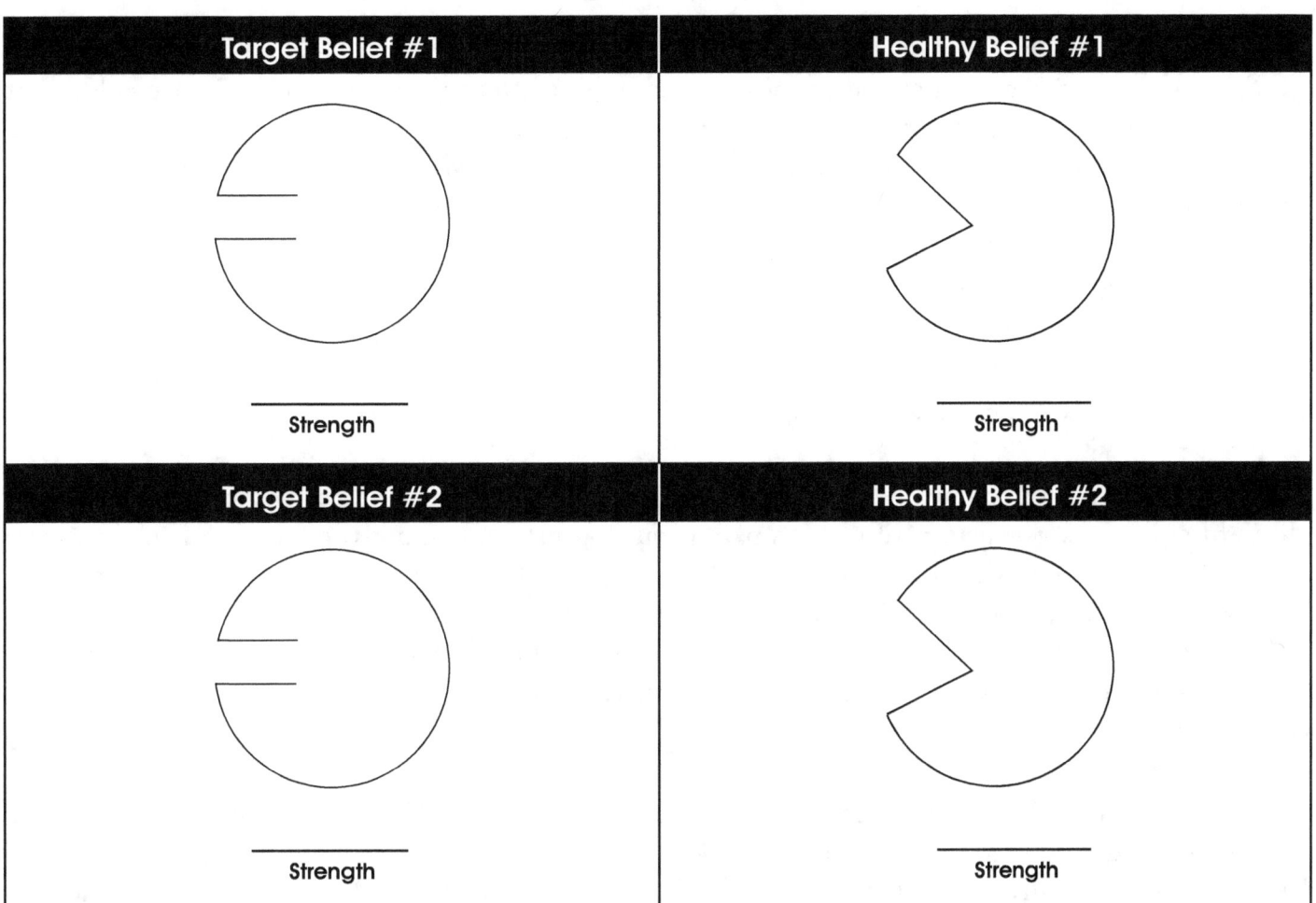

Tool #9: Evidence Logs

Here is where the hard work begins! This is a tool you will use throughout your treatment, regardless of what other tools you may be using and at what stage of treatment you may be at. This is the tough, tough work of gradually working to develop your healthy belief. How do we change beliefs, anyway? It's a difficult process, no doubt. What we need to do is to *reexamine historical evidence*, *get better at noticing current evidence* **and** *intentionality initiate ongoing experiences around which to create new evidence.*

Think of any belief that you have changed over time in any area of your life. Maybe you used to not believe in God and now you do. Perhaps you used to not believe in global warming and now you do. Maybe you used to believe in life on other planets and now you don't. For example, I have a client who is a marine biology major in college – his chief interest is in Megalodon sharks, which he was initially convinced were not extinct. After a lot of scientific research, he now no longer believes that. Did you used to hold more conservative political beliefs, and your beliefs are now more progressive? You get the gist. You can use a belief that you have changed in any area of life to illustrate this process. How do

beliefs change? By examining the evidence created by experience and the meaning that we assign to it.

Take a belief many people once held. (WARNING! UPCOMING CONTENT NOT APPROPRIATE FOR KIDS!) Santa Claus is not real. If you believed in his existence when you were six years old, what was the "evidence" that supported your belief? He brought presents. They said "from Santa" on the wrapping. He drank the milk that was set out for him. He knew what presents were desired from the letters that was sent to him at the North Pole. The local weather even tracks him on the Doppler radar!

Over time, most people reexamine the pieces of evidence and assign new meaning to them. By doing so, they change their belief.

But they have to *experience* new evidence.

Some children recognize Papa beneath the Santa suit and false white beard. Some children stay up all night and sneak downstairs to catch a parent putting presents under the tree. Some children are observant enough to notice that "Santa" has Mommy's identical hand writing or wrapping paper. The child who does *not* go out of their way to look for these things holds onto the old, false belief much longer because they are not looking for evidence to the contrary. In fact, when I myself was becoming suspicious but desperately wanted to believe that he was real as a child, I began actively searching out confirmation of his existence.

In the same way, for any of us to change our beliefs, we must be *willing* to examine evidence fairly. We are naturally (consciously or unconsciously) looking for evidence to support our existing belief. But we must be equally willing to consider evidence to the contrary as well. This is what the evidence logs do: they provide a tool to facilitate *purposefully looking for evidence* to support the new belief you are attempting to construct. If your current unhealthy belief is that you are a failure, then you are purposefully looking for evidence that you can succeed. For some cognitive behavioral therapy (CBT) exercises, we will ask people to log evidence on *both* sides. But because people with PDs have such deeply engrained beliefs, their natural tendency will be to see only evidence that supports the current belief. So, for the purpose of this exercise, it is important to use the right column only to log evidence that supports the belief. The left column will remain blank.

As you record the evidence, think about how it felt to have that experience. As you do, ask yourself: *In this moment* how much do I believe _____ and how much do I believe _____?
  (unhealthy belief)   (healthy belief)

Remember, you will inherently *not notice* evidence that will be helpful because your filter is directing you away from it, so be vigilant. Also, when you log evidence for a healthy belief, you will get that little voice in your head that says, "but… it doesn't count because of this or that." Go ahead and record the evidence anyway even if you have trouble believing it at the time.

Log the believability rating as you record each piece of evidence. Note that these numbers will go up

and down, because beliefs fluctuate. But over time, watch your unhealthy numbers generally trend down and your healthy numbers trend up. The more they change, the more balanced your lenses will be come and you will get your "buttons pushed" less frequently!

Look at the example below. Then begin completing your own evidence log, working on one belief at a time. When you have more than one icebergs to conquer, the more effort you put into chiseling one at a time, the more progress you will make.

Example: Evidence Log

Unhealthy Belief: 90%   Healthy Belief: 10%

Date	"Unrelenting Standards"	% Belief	"Doesn't Have to be Perfect/exact"	% Belief
7/14		80%	Left work in middle of a project	20%
7/16		85%	Only enough gas to fill three quarters of my tank	15%
7/17		85%	Couldn't get the edge sawed off my woodworking project	15%
7/18		80%	Couldn't park straight due to another car in the spot next to me	20%
7/20		78%	Light switches are both up at the same time	22%

Conclusions: I am getting a little better with things being off—I am realizing I may need to err on the side of sloppy to be normal.

My Evidence Log

Unhealthy Belief: **Healthy Belief:**

Date		% Belief		% Belief

Conclusions _____

_____

Tool #10: Productivity Planner Tool

High performers are often task-oriented individuals. That is, many of them gain a sense of fulfillment by accomplishing projects and mastering tasks. A good day entails "getting a lot done." There are a thousand courses out there devoted to time management, but the reality is there is nothing new under the sun. We all have the same 168 hours in a week and each of us gets to choose how we spend them. Gordon McDonald jokes in his book *Ordering Your Private World*, "Has anybody seen my time? I think I've lost it!" Being intentional about how we spend our time is one of the most important keys to success. And what is success, anyway? Well, we each define that concept differently. So it is important to prioritize our time each day according to our own values: whatever is most important to us. This might involve faith, family, friends, income, education, charitable causes, or whatever you believe to be important in life. We all have things we "have to" accomplish in life as well (pay bills, feed our children, etc.).

The following simple tool is a way to help you be intentional about how you spend each day. Many of the world's most successful people plan weeks, months, and even years out in advance. This doesn't mean they leave no room for flexibility or spontaneity, but it does likely mean that all of us would benefit from taking a bigger-picture look at how we are prioritizing our time. Use this tool to devise a plan to get your "have to's," i.e., your duties, done, but also put plans in place to accomplish your dreams and live your life in the most fulfilling way possible. And remember not to prioritize your schedule… instead, schedule your priorities. There is a BIG difference! Best wishes in taking charge of your life in a more productive and meaningful way.

See next page for *Productivity Planner* tool

Priorities Duties

	Monday		Tuesday		Wednesday		Thursday		Friday		Saturday		Sunday	
	Planned	Active	Planned	Active	Planned	Active	Planned	Active	Planned	Active	Planned	Active	Planned	Active
6 AM														
7 AM														
8 AM														
9 AM														
10 AM														
11 AM														
12 PM														
1 PM														
2 PM														
3 PM														
4 PM														
5 PM														
6 PM														

Tool #11: Progress, Not Perfection Tool

As previously mentioned, failure beliefs are common in perfectionists. If a person believes, "If I can't do something perfectly, it's not worth doing at all," it makes sense that they overwork themselves; on the other hand, for some, it can be difficult to push oneself to do anything that they can later feel good about. Since the perfectionist never accomplishes anything "good enough," they cannot give themselves credit for the progress they make. This can actually reinforce the failure belief or the negative self-image that drives many problematic behaviors in that person. Thus, it can be helpful to *be intentionally mindful of small steps of progress* and ensure that proper credit is given where due. Some find it helpful to place message cards with the phrase, "Progress not Perfection" (or some other related phrase that resonates) in spots where their perfectionism tends to manifest worst, like their workdesk. You may have heard it said—and it's true—that perfection is the enemy of excellence!

Use the following log to help yourself monitor small steps of progress in key areas of your life.

Example:

Issue	"Perfection"	Where I Started	Progress
Cleaning out garage	Whole garage picked up, swept, and mopped	Eight hours ago, it was a "complete mess"	Eight hours of work, can now fit one car in the two-car garage

- Things I can do this week to make progress toward my goal:
    1. Clean off workbench
    2. Organize automotive supplies
    3. Label Chemicals

My "Progress, not Perfection" Charts

Issue	"Perfection"	Where I Started	Progress

- Things I can do this week to make progress toward my goal

    1. _____
    2. _____
    3. _____

Issue	"Perfection"	Where I Started	Progress

- Things I can do this week to make progress toward my goal

    1. _____
    2. _____
    3. _____

Tool #12: Tolerating Distress

Due to the high standards people with OCPD have, distress is a frequent occurrence and usually takes the outward form of annoyance.

When one's past involves constantly being evaluated, corrected, scolded, criticized, or worse, over time, this message of one being "not good enough" leads to the internalization of the belief that one should be perfect. The desire to meet high standards or to achieve goals is healthy; but the desire to be perfect is unhealthy. No human being is perfect. Thus, believing we "should" be is setting ourselves up for stress, depression, anger, and ultimately, failure. Along the way, this way of thinking can put us in a state of ongoing and persistent distress. Hopefully you have (and/or will) learn some skills for alleviating the distress. But since this is not possible in all situations, rather than reacting in a way that is counterproductive, it can also be helpful to have some tools in your toolbox for tolerating the distress until you can eliminate it completely.

Peruse the following list of skill categories that can be used to tolerate distress. Use them to formulate a collection of strategies that you can add to your personal toolbox for the purpose of not acting on emotions which you temporarily cannot overcome.

Distraction Techniques. A distraction technique might be defined as any coping skill that inherently requires thought. For instance, taking a hot bath is a good skill for some people in some situations, but it is possible to sit in the tub, stare at the tiled wall, and continue to stew in a way that gets one worked up. So we would not define it as a distraction technique. Reading, on the other hand, can get a person's mind so immersed in the written material that while their mind is "somewhere else," their emotional arousal temporarily subsides. The following are examples of distraction techniques. Put an "X" by the skills you could see yourself potentially using.

- ❏ Read a book, article, or blog
- ❏ Count to one hundred forwards and then backwards
- ❏ Recite as many states (or comparable regions in your country) as you can
- ❏ Sing a song
- ❏ Watch a movie
- ❏ Memorize or recite a meaningful passage
- ❏ Call a friend and talk about anything other than what you are annoyed with
- ❏ Listen to a podcast
- ❏ Do guided imagery
- ❏ Learn (and practice) deep breathing
- ❏ Think about the worst moment in your life. Compare it to what you are dealing with in this moment.
- ❏ Choose to put it off. If you believe you must stew, pick a time later in the day.
- ❏ Go for a walk/run. Purposefully focus on your surroundings as you go.

Draw from the list on the previous, or come up with your own, to tolerate distress when you start to notice it rising up in your body.

My Distress Tolerance Skills

1. _____
2. _____
3. _____
4. _____
5. _____

Tool #13: Delegation Tool

Due to being bothered by others' lower standards or their "not doing things good enough," perfectionists often have difficulty delegating. The inability to delegate can lead to difficulty completing projects, poor leadership, and upsetting other people (who perceive you as critical). Use the following tool to assess whether this is a problem for you, and if so, to identify areas to work on it. This tool will ask you to identify people in three different areas of your life with whom you interact regularly and to ask each of them to point out areas in which you could delegate, in order to practice refuting thoughts which are keeping you from moving forward, and taking concrete action steps.

Person	Areas of Suggested Delegation	My Automatic Thought	My Rational Response
Person # 1			
Person # 2			
Person # 3			

- One thing I agree to delegate this week _____

_____

- When I delegate it, I am likely to feel _____

_____

- To cope with those feelings, rather than choose to do the task myself, I will

_____

_____

Tool #14: Accept Reality

Those with OCPD and other perfectionistic people engage in a lot of "should" thinking toward others and the world. You may remember that "should" statements are distorted because they have nothing to do with reality. They have only to do with the way we think things should be (or ought to be, or must be, or need to be, or supposed to be, or any of those other "should" in disguise). Thus, refusal to accept some aspect of reality keeps people stuck in those emotions within the anger family. By the way, accepting reality doesn't mean there is never a time to in response to feelings of anger or annoyance—, although, if you have OCPD or other perfectionistic tendencies, it is likely you are doing or saying things more often than is in your best interest. But to the extent that we can acknowledge that "it is what it is" (i.e., we accept a reality), the easier it will be for us to act in an effective way if we choose to.

Consider the following example and then complete some "accept reality" exercises on your own. Again, these usually do not help significantly the first few times, but, almost everyone who persists at this tool improves significantly over time.

Example:

Date: 7/11

- Event that Triggered Annoyance

    The spreadsheet my team member completed was slightly misaligned to the left.

- What are some of the "should" statements going through my mind?
    - "This should be straight."
    - "Since it isn't, it looks unprofessional."
    - "Maybe I should stay and redo it."

- Frustration/Anger Level (0-10)

    5

- What are the realities of this situation I need to accept in order to feel better?
    - "He did it, not me."
    - "I can't clock any more overtime."
    - "My wife is waiting on me at home."
    - "This is only an internal document anyway; nobody outside the company will see it."
    - "The numbers on the report are accurate. That's what really counts."

- New Frustration/Anger Level (0-10)

    4

- Action Plan: I will use the following three skills to cope
    1. Leave the building immediately. It's time to go home.
    2. Call my sister and talk to her about holiday plans while I leave. That will get my mind on something else.
    3. Let it go. If my mind returns to this issue, focus on the benefit—I will be home on time for once!

My "Accepting Reality" Log

Date: _____

- Event that Triggered Annoyance _____
  _____
  _____

- What are some of the "should" statements" going through my mind? _____
  _____
  _____
  _____

- Frustration/Anger Level (0-10) _____

- What are the realities of this situation I need to accept to feel better? _____
  _____
  _____
  _____

- New Frustration/Anger Level (0-10) _____

- Action Plan _____
  _____
  _____
  _____

- I will use the following three skills to cope

    1. _____

    2. _____

    3. _____

Tool #15: Develop Compassion

Compassion oozes from some people, but typically not from those who are also perfectionists. Why? First off, as was previously mentioned, people with this trait are often more task oriented than people oriented. This doesn't mean they don't like people or can't be nice individuals; but in their minds, getting the job done always takes precedent over people's feelings ("If somebody gets hurt along the way, that's just too bad, but the important thing is that the job gets done.") Task-oriented people reading this are probably thinking, "Yes, that's about right," while people-oriented people are likely thinking, "What a jerk!"

Perfectionists aren't "mean" people. But everyone has their strengths and weaknesses, and an area for potential growth for all task-oriented people is that of demonstrating compassion. Specifically, because perfectionists have that "unrelenting standards" schema, they can often be perceived as overly critical by others. And they not only have the tendency to be overly critical of others, but they can have the tendency to be harsh on themselves as well. Thus, developing compassion is a vital skill for perfectionists to work at. Beating people up (emotionally) is no way to win friends and improve your own self-esteem!

Compassion can be difficult to develop: It requires patience; it requires the ability to cut yourself and others some slack; it calls for empathy (the ability to step out of one's shoes and into the shoes of someone else.)

Use the following tool to help cultivate softer feelings toward yourself or someone who bothers you.

Compassion Tool

- A person I find myself being critical of _____

- Three things I have in common with them

    1. _____

    2. _____

    3. _____

- What could be going on in their life that could be contributing to them acting the way they do? _____

_____

_____

_____

- When I picture that person as a small child, I feel (hint: if it is myself I am working on compassion towards, it can help to find an old picture of myself from my childhood) _____

_____

_____

_____

- One song that evokes feelings of compassion and concern for me

_____

- One time I saw or heard someone else treat an animal or small child poorly. Describe my thoughts and feelings _____

_____

_____

_____

- When I hear that critical voice in my head, I will _____

- One trait I like about that person _____

Chapter 2: The Obsessive Compulsive Personality Disorder

- One time someone showed compassion toward me when I didn't "deserve" it _____
_____
_____

- One thing I find pleasurable in life _____
_____

- Three things/people that make me laugh
    1. _____
    2. _____
    3. _____

- One way I could show kindness toward that person _____
_____
_____
_____

CHAPTER 3: THE AVOIDANT PERSONALITY DISORDER

The Avoidant Personality Disorder

Hidden agenda: To not be hurt emotionally or judged

Prevalence rates: Approximately 3% of the general population

Gender distribution: Equally diagnosed in men and women

Cognitive profile:

- View of self: "I am vulnerable," "I am socially inept," "I am inferior"

- View of others: "Others are critical," "Others are demeaning/rejecting"

- View of world: "The world will reject me"

Common schemas: Approval seeking, social isolation, emotional inhibition

Common cognitive distortions: Rationalization, mind reading, fortune telling, magnification, personalization

Overdeveloped traits: Avoidance, inhibition

Underdeveloped traits: Self-assertion, gregariousness

Whom they date/marry: Nobody (but they'd like to)

Where they work: Truck drivers, independent copy editors

Other Random Nuggets:

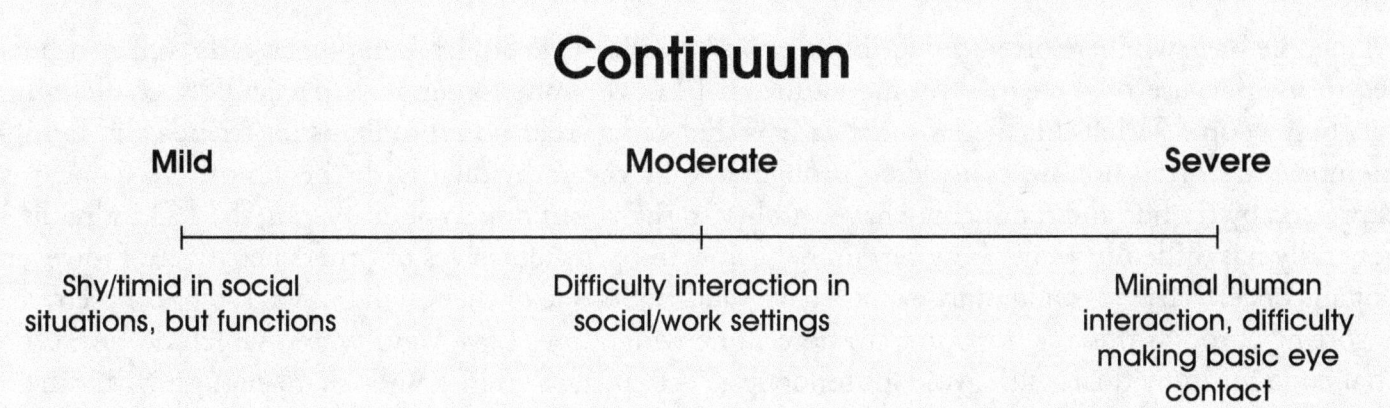

Tool #1: Trait Checklist

Individuals that suffer from the characteristics of avoidant personality disorder (APD) have a number of commonalities. Whether you are a loved one has this full blown condition, or some of the traits of it, survey the following checklist. The more of these you check yes to, the more likely it is this pattern of behavior is causing some problems occupationally, relationally, or socially.

- ❏ Excessively shy
- ❏ Has few friends
- ❏ Unwilling to get involved socially if they are not absolutely certain the other person likes them
- ❏ Preoccupied with being rejected
- ❏ Is almost certain others will hurt them (emotionally)
- ❏ Won't start new relationships due to believing they are inadequate
- ❏ Seeks out employment with little interpersonal interaction
- ❏ Even the slightest criticism produces intense hurt
- ❏ If somebody dislikes them, it is the end of the world
- ❏ Gets angry when asked overly "personal" questions

Tool #2: Expressions of Concern

All people have what are often called "blind spots": qualities we don't see in ourselves as well as others see in us. Because of the ego-syntonic nature of PDs, this phenomenon is particularly challenging for these people. What this means practically is that things that pose problems for friends and family members are often not are considered problematic by the individual with the condition. Concerns expressed by friends and family may have validity to them, but due to poor insight, the PD individual generally has difficulty seeing how certain behaviors impact themselves or others negatively. However, not all concerns friends and family express have validity. So, one of the tough but vital steps for recovery is sorting through these "complaints" to determine which ones have validity and which do not. One challenge for individuals with avoidant tendencies is that they often do not share enough with others for them to form an accurate idea of what is really going on with them.

Use the following tool to identify *who* has expressed concern, *what* the exact concerns are, and *why* they see them as potentially hurtful. Look at the example, then complete your own and answer the questions that follow.

Example:

Person Expressing Concern	Action Causing Concern	Reason for Concern
1. Tori (classmate)	1. Not showing up for class group projects	1. Might not pass course, might not graduate from program
2. Julie (friend)	2. Not socializing	2. Never make friends, date, or be happy in life
3. Sister (Angela)	3. Not coming to family functions	3. Getting depressed

Questions:

- Who are three people I trust to "shoot straight" with me, by whom I can run these concerns to get their opinion?

    1. Aunt

    2. ?

    3. ?

- With which concerns can I at least see where the person is coming from?

    I do not make friends easily

- Which concerns can I see the most validity in?

    I do want to get married and have kids some day

- I am willing to take the following steps to change one of the concerns:

    1. Keep my appointments

    2. Come to Christmas for at least a few hours

    3. Go to the next group activity for class this Thursday

My Expressions of Concern

Person Expressing Concern	Action Causing Concern	Reason for Concern
1.	1.	1.
2.	2.	2.
3.	3.	3.
4.	4.	4.
5.	5.	5.

Questions:

- Who are three people I trust to "shoot straight" with me, by whom I can run these concerns by to get their opinion?

    1. _____

    2. _____

    3. _____

- With which concerns can I at least see where the person is coming from? _____
_____
_____

- Which concerns can I see the most validity in? _____
_____
_____

- I am willing to take the following steps to change one of the concerns
    1. _____
    2. _____
    3. _____

Tool #3: Pros and Cons

This tool helps you evaluate the potential pros and cons of your avoidant behaviors. It is called a *four-box pros and cons*. Sometimes it can be beneficial to look at not only the advantages and disadvantages of maintaining certain behaviors but also the advantages and disadvantages of changing them. After listing the pros and cons of each, it can be even more helpful to rate, on a scale of 0-10, how important each item is. Consider the example that is provided. Then complete one on your own!

Example: Pros and Cons of Avoiding Behavior

Pros of Remaining Avoidant	Pros of Facing my Fears
Won't ever be embarrassed (7)	I could get some friends (10)
Won't be rejected by a man/woman (10)	I could meet a special guy/girl (10)
Won't hurt anyone's feelings (8)	I could have more fun in life (8)
Cons of Remaining Avoidant	**Cons of Facing my Fears**
I stay lonely (9)	I'll be uncomfortable (6)

Results:

__25__ Reasons to remain avoidant

__28__ Reasons to face my fears

__9__ Reasons to not remain avoidant

__6__ Reasons to not face my fears

My Conclusions: My fear of being lonely forever is finally starting to overcome my fear of getting hurt

My Commitment:

1. Go to one meet up group this week

2. Say yes to my friend's invitation to come over Saturday

My Pros and Cons of Avoiding Behavior

Pros of Remaining Avoidant	Pros of Facing my Fears

Cons of Remaining Avoidant	Cons of Facing my Fears

Results:

_____ Reasons to remain avoidant

_____ Reasons to face my fears

_____ Reasons to not remain avoidant

_____ Reasons to not face my fears

My Conclusions _____
_____
_____
_____

My Commitment(s) _____
_____
_____
_____
_____

Tool #4: Identify Behavioral Targets

Avoidance manifests differently in different people. Some behaviors include shutting down in relationships (while harboring anger toward the person), limiting employment opportunities so as to not be around people, never taking chances to meet new friends, avoiding having tough conversations, and more.

Use this tool to identify some of your avoidant behaviors that you or others have noticed. Feel free to use any of the above behaviors that fit, or list some of your own.

- Behaviors related to my avoidance traits that I or someone else identified which I am willing to target to improve my situation

    1. _____
    2. _____
    3. _____
    4. _____
    5. _____

Tool #5: Intimacy Circles

Intimacy is a scary word for a lot of people. If the sound of it makes you cringe, this exercise is definitely for you—and even if it doesn't, this exercise likely will still benefit you. It will benefit almost everyone in some way. Why? Because almost everyone could benefit from improving at least one interpersonal relationship in their life. Some people's lives could be enriched with more friends. Others need to learn to set boundaries with someone in their life. A lot of people have "trust issues." Yet others would be happier in life if they learned to pick healthier people to date or form friendships with; toxic people have a way of draining people of their energy and joy. A certain percentage of the population would be much less prone to mood swings if they could be okay alone. Some would find more fulfillment in life if they could share more with people in their lives; others would not be hurt as often if they learned to share less with those in their life. A lot of people walk around with their "walls" up. Some have difficulty expressing feelings. Some have been accused of being too "needy." Others have difficulty asking for help.

You may have heard intimacy defined as "Into-Me-See"——the degree to which we let people see into us, and vice versa. A lot of my clients have found this "play on words" to be a helpful way to remember its definition and connotations.

Use the following tool to evaluate the relationships in your life. Use the percentage signs to help you decide which people to put in which circles. No other person goes in the ME circle (though some people choose to put God here). This is for you alone. People who belong in circle #1 are those with whom you would feel comfortable sharing ANY problem in life, no matter how personal (a sexual problem, something related to an abusive situation, a salary issue, etc.). People in circle #2 are those in your life with whom there may be a personal issue or two (like the ones mentioned above) that you would not share, but you would be comfortable sharing ALMOST anything (roughly 75%) about your life. People in circle #3 may get about half of your personal stuff, but the other half you probably would not trust them with. People in circle #4 would be your very casual relationships. Maybe they know whether you are married or where you work or something of that nature, but you don't share very much with them (roughly 25%). And people in circle #5 get nothing. For some people, these are individuals

whom they have just met, so they could be candidates to move closer in as they get to know them. Or, these are people who at one point in life were closer in, but they have done something to violate trust, so they have had to be moved out one or more rings.

Relationships are challenging for all people with PDs or traits of PDs, but avoidant individuals' only trigger is RELATIONSHIPS. So, this exercise can seem overwhelming. But this is where the most powerful work will happen for you if you are in this PD group. Gradually identify the people who are least threatening to start your work with, and then go from there. Take your time. But face your fears! This is where you genuinely grow.

Keep these ideas in mind as you consider who truly belongs where as you complete your circles. Your first task is to think about all the people in your life and where they go in your circles. Then consider the questions that follow to get you started making healthy changes to your relationships. Work with your therapist or other helping professional if you need ongoing guidance or accountability.

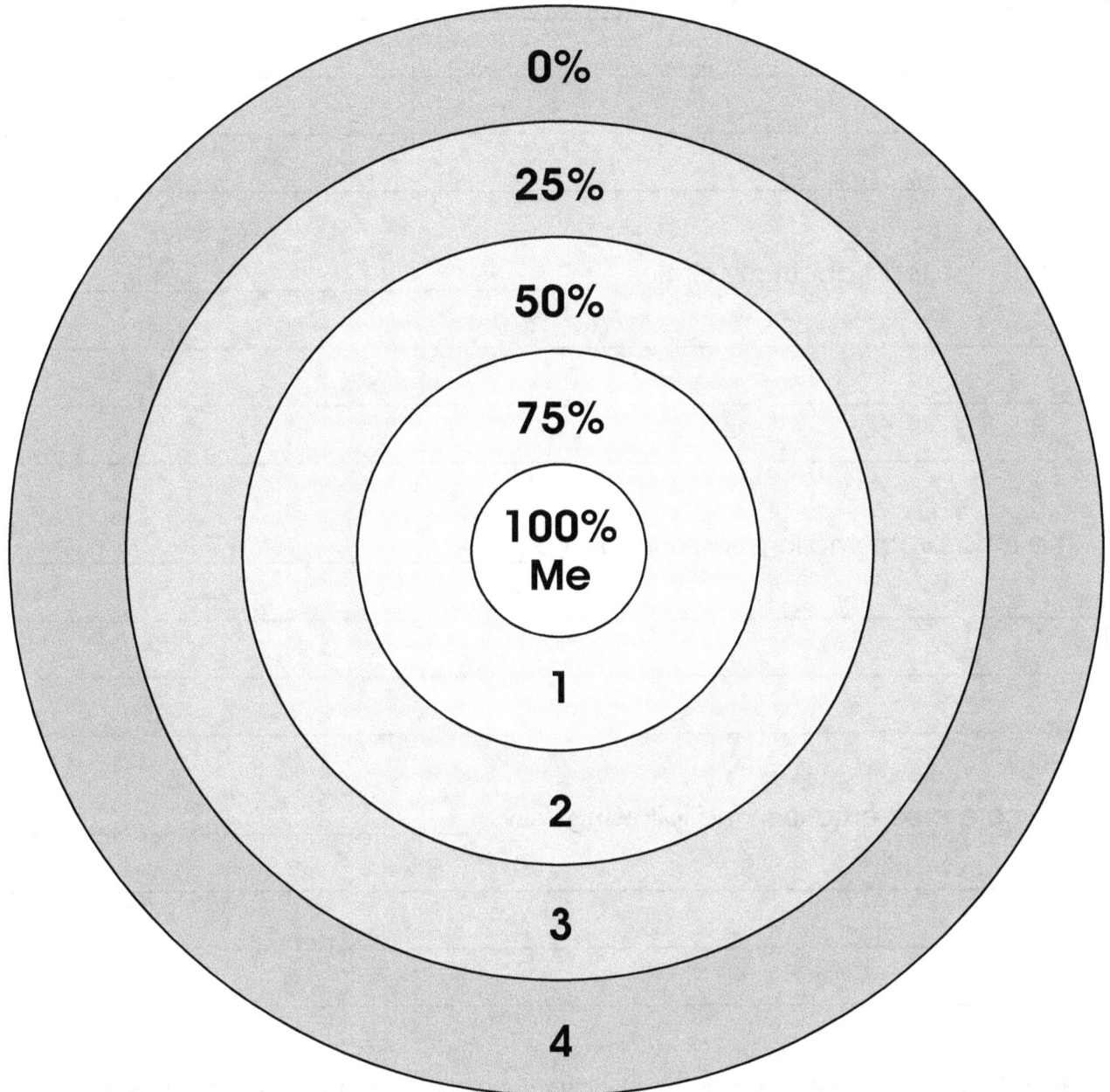

Intimacy Circles Follow-Up Starter Questions

- General observations about my circles _____
_____
_____
_____

- What I like most about my circles _____
_____
_____
_____

- What I like least about my circles _____
_____
_____
_____

- The most problematic people in my life _____
_____
_____
_____

- They are problematic in the following ways _____
_____
_____
_____

- People in my life whose opinions I actually care about and on a scale of 0-10 how much I care what they think _____
_____
_____
_____

- People in my life whose opinions I don't care about _____
_____
_____

- People in my life whom I have hurt/violated/taken advantage of _____
  _____
  _____
  _____

- People in my life who have moved themselves out in my circles due to my behavior
  _____
  _____
  _____
  _____
  _____

- I could improve my circles if I were willing to keep the following rules (which I have not previously been willing to keep) _____
  _____
  _____
  _____
  _____

- One step I will take TODAY to improve my relationship circles _____
  _____
  _____
  _____
  _____

Tool #6: Identify and Restructure Automatic Thoughts

A staple component of treatment for any psychological condition is recognizing the thought processes that are driving the problem behaviors and maintaining the symptoms. In colloquial language, you may hear this referred to as "self-talk." To speak in the terms of the Mark Twain quote in the introduction ("If all you have is a hammer, everything looks like a nail"): This is the "hammer." While treatment of personality disorders requires more tools than just a hammer, the hammer is still a useful tool to have in your toolbox.

Some people develop an awareness of their thoughts and get better at noticing them, but do nothing to change them. For example, if we recognize that we are overweight, but do nothing to change our diets

or exercise levels, we will stay overweight. In the same way, if we recognize thoughts that are driving problem behavior but do nothing to change them, our symptoms are likely to remain.

So, one cognitive tool you can use is what is called challenging distorted thoughts when you recognize them. Refer to the beginning of this chapter for some distorted thoughts common in avoidant personality disorder. *"Challenging,"* in this case, basically means "arguing" with the specific content of the thoughts. There are a number of techniques that can be used for doing this, including looking at evidence, seeking input from others, researching the facts, considering past or possible future results, or good old-fashioned logic, just to name a few.

The following tool asks you to identify specific avoidant thoughts that enter your mind, challenge them in some way, and if you want to, rate your challenge on a scale of 0-10, indicating how meaningful the challenge is. Take a look at the example, and then do one on your own. This may be a tool that you will benefit from using on an ongoing basis.

Example: Thought Log

Avoidant Thought	Rational Responses
It is okay to lie to him because he might judge me if he found out, and he has no right to know where I am at anyway	Lying is against my values - I don't like to lie for any reason
	He might not judge me if he knew - he does similar things, after all
	Even if he judged me, I don't have to have his approval for everything I do
	I would feel uncomfortable telling him, but then I would have nothing to hide
	I probably should tell him more than I do now if I am really going to marry him - as my fiancé, he probably has a right to know more than I've told him

Analysis: This thirty-eight-year-old woman recently accepted a marriage proposal from a guy she had been dating for six months, due to a burning desire to have children and a fear that her "biological clock is ticking." She is still uncomfortable disclosing most personal details to him and gets very defensive when he asks her questions. She withholds much of what she does from him and avoids every question related to her whereabouts or even how she spends her days while he is at work. She is capable of generating some useful rational responses, although early in treatment her motivations for avoiding remain strong. It is a good sign, however, that she is capable of generating several challenges that she at least believes at the intellectual level. Much of ongoing treatment will emphasize internalizing these ideas.

My Avoidant Thought Log

Avoidant Thought	Rational Responses

Tool #7: Historical Experiences Worksheet

As with most, if not all, personality disorders, it is believed that there are multiple pathways to avoidant personality disorder. There is little research as to the causes of APD. Genetic factors are believed to be less influential in this PD than others. Peruse the following historical experiences worksheet and put an "X" beside factors that were a part of your experiences from a young age.

- ❑ Parents who got angry if emotions were expressed
- ❑ Disagreement was always met with conflict
- ❑ Was criticized (or felt a perception of criticism) often
- ❑ Parents emphasized *"quiet obedience"*
- ❑ Got feelings hurt often
- ❑ Had one or more significant figure in their life that was (at least perceived as) judgmental

- Describe how the experiences checked above apply specifically to you and the impact you believe they continue to have in your life today

_____
_____
_____
_____
_____
_____
_____
_____
_____
_____

Tool #8: Belief Identification

As has been discussed, all behaviors are a product of beliefs. Beliefs drive behavior. Due to the compelling nature of beliefs in individuals with PDs, these deeper-level beliefs often have to be modified to help create lasting change. As noted at the beginning of this chapter, common beliefs in people with APD include approval seeking, social isolation, and emotional inhibition, among others. Review their definitions if you don't have them fresh in your mind. Get with your therapist. Include friends and family who are willing to give you feedback. Identify one or two beliefs that you believe drive your target behaviors to work on in treatment. Write them inside Judy Beck's "Pac-Man" visual aid (which was explained in the introduction).

Target Belief # 1	Target Belief #2
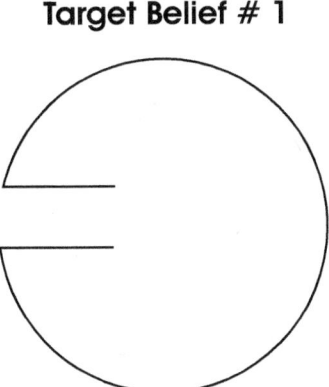	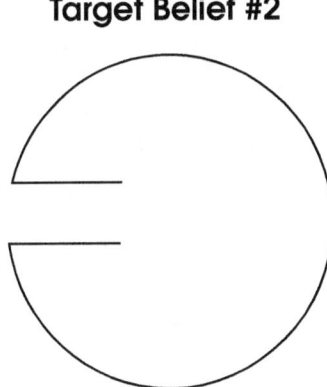

Beliefs always come in pairs. For every maladaptive (or unhealthy) belief we possess, we also possess an alternate, adaptive (or healthy) belief. For instance, even though an individual may have the belief, "I must isolate myself because I am a social outcast," they also have the belief, however faint, "I can fit in."

I have given you the "pushing buttons" language, the "Pac-Man" visual, and the "filters" imagery. Here is another representation which I hope helps illustrate the point: We could think of beliefs as lenses. For people who wear glasses, this visual probably comes fairly intuitively. Healthier individuals are able to engage in more balanced information processing. Figuratively speaking they are able to see out of both the left and the right "lenses" equally. This is the goal of belief modification work: balanced information processing. In other words, to be able to see both sides objectively and to be able to recognize when they fail or make mistakes, so they can learn from them; and also to be able to acknowledge when they succeed and be able to take a compliment. Although nobody is perfect and everyone has their biases, healthier people's lenses are closer to the 50/50 range (50% failure/50% success). Before treatment, people with PDs, due to their more compelling beliefs, often start with numbers such as 99%/1%. ***Intentional and sustained effort*** is required to create a healthier belief balance.

So, now that you have identified your unhealthy beliefs driving your target behaviors, identify in your own words what you would call the opposite, healthy belief. Write it in the opposite belief structure that the "triangle" could fit into.

After you have identified your one or two healthy and unhealthy beliefs, ask yourself: "What percentage of the time do I believe the unhealthy belief? What percentage of the time do I believe the healthy belief?" Write your numbers in the line next to each belief (they should total 100%). Then you are ready to move on to Tool #9!

See the example first, and then do one on your own!

Example: Belief Identification

Target Belief #1	Healthy Belief #1
"I am an outsider" — 95% Strength	"I can fit in" — 5% Strength
Target Belief #2	**Healthy Belief #2**
Strength	Strength

My Beliefs

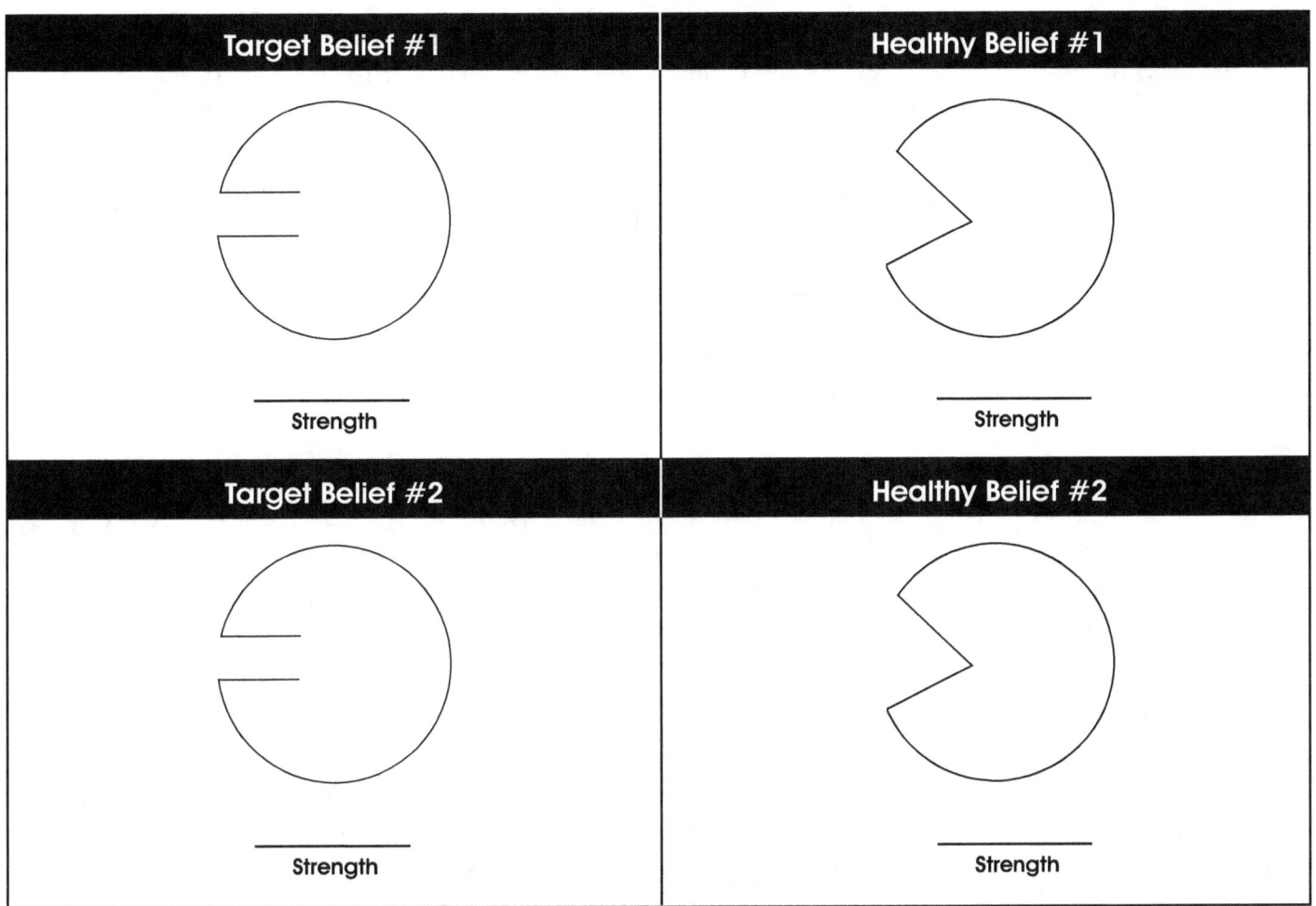

Tool #9: Evidence Logs

Here is where the hard work begins! This is a tool you will use throughout your treatment, regardless of what other tools you may be using and at what stage of treatment you may be at. This is the tough, tough work of gradually working to develop your healthy belief. How do we change beliefs, anyway? It's a difficult process, no doubt. What we need to do is to *reexamine historical evidence, get better at noticing current evidence* **and** *intentionality initiate ongoing experiences around which to create new evidence.*

Think of any belief that you have changed over time in any area of your life. Maybe you used to not believe in God and now you do. Perhaps you used to not believe in global warming and now you do. Maybe you used to believe in life on other planets and now you don't. For example, I have a client who is a marine biology major in college – his chief interest is in Megalodon sharks, which he was initially convinced were not extinct. After a lot of scientific research, he now no longer believes that. Did you used to hold more conservative political beliefs, and your beliefs are now more progressive? You get the gist. You can use a belief that you have changed in *any* area of life to illustrate this process. How do

beliefs change? By examining the evidence created by experience and the meaning that we assign to it.

Take a belief many people once held. (WARNING! UPCOMING CONTENT NOT APPROPRIATE FOR KIDS!) Santa Claus is not real. If you believed in his existence when you were six years old, what was the "evidence" that supported your belief? He brought presents. They said "from Santa" on the wrapping. He drank the milk that was set out for him. He knew what presents were desired from the letters that was sent to him at the North Pole. The local weather even tracks him on the Doppler radar!

Over time, most people reexamine the pieces of evidence and assign new meaning to them. By doing so, they change their belief.

But they have to *experience* new evidence.

Some children recognize Papa beneath the Santa suit and false white beard. Some children stay up all night and sneak downstairs to catch a parent putting presents under the tree. Some children are observant enough to notice that "Santa" has Mommy's identical hand writing or wrapping paper. The child who *does not go out of their way to look for these things* holds onto the old, false belief much longer because they are not looking for evidence to the contrary. In fact, when I myself was becoming suspicious but desperately wanted to believe that he was real as a child, I began actively searching out confirmation of his existence.

In the same way, for any of us to change our beliefs, we must be *willing* to examine evidence fairly. We are naturally (consciously or unconsciously) looking for evidence to support our existing belief. But we must be equally willing to consider evidence to the contrary as well. This is what the evidence logs do: they provide a tool to facilitate *purposefully looking for evidence* to support the new belief you are attempting to construct. If your current unhealthy belief is that you are a failure, then you are purposefully looking for evidence that you can succeed. For some cognitive behavioral therapy (CBT) exercises, we will ask people to log evidence on *both* sides. But because people with PDs have such deeply engrained beliefs, their natural tendency will be to see only evidence that supports the current belief. So, for the purpose of this exercise, it is important to use the right column only to log evidence that supports the belief. The left column will remain blank.

As you record the evidence, think about how it felt to have that experience. As you do, ask yourself: *In this moment* how much do I believe _____ and how much do I believe _____?

                                              (unhealthy belief)   (healthy belief)

Remember, you will inherently *not notice* evidence that will be helpful because your filter is directing you away from it, so be vigilant. Also, when you log evidence for a healthy belief, you will get that little voice in your head that says, "but… it doesn't count because of this or that." Go ahead and record the evidence anyway even if you have trouble believing it at the time.

Log the believability rating as you record each piece of evidence. Note that these numbers will go up

and down, because beliefs fluctuate. But over time, watch your unhealthy numbers generally trend down and your healthy numbers trend up. The more they change, the more balanced your lenses will be come and you will get your "buttons pushed" less frequently!

Look at the example below. Then begin completing your own evidence log, working on one belief at a time. When you have more than one icebergs to conquer, the more effort you put into chiseling one at a time, the more progress you will make.

Example: Evidence Log

Unhealthy Belief: 95% Healthy Belief: 5%

Date	"I am an outsider"	% Belief	"I can fit in"	% Belief
3/12		94%	Looked up some groups online with similar hobbies; it helped a bit to see others doing some of the things I like	6%
3/13		94%	Shared something with my cousin that I never had before	6%
3/14		95%	Invited Suzie to come into my apartment for the first time	5%
3/18		93%	Accompanied my friend to her reading club	7%
3/19		90%	Went to a knitting group, where the leader made me feel as comfortable as I ever have around strangers	10%

Conclusions: I am still VERY uncomfortable. But it does at least help to see there are people that I might have a little bit in common with.

My Evidence Log

Unhealthy Belief: **Healthy Belief:**

Date		% Belief		% Belief

Conclusions _____

_____

Tool #10: Identification and Expression of Emotions

This may seem simplistic to some people, but one of the biggest difficulties for individuals with APD is identifying and expressing feelings. Sometimes they know what their feelings but choose not to express it for some of the reasons above generally, so as not to get their feelings hurt. Refusal to express feelings honestly is a common safety behavior with APD. Many actually go significantly out of their way to not feel certain emotions; and, some have done this to the extent that they have become numb and honestly don't know how they are feeling. Many were never given a language for expressing emotion nor the skills to convey them to others.

Use this tool to 1) identify emotions that you feel most frequently, and 2) consider the people in your life to whom you may need to express them.

Put an "X" by the feelings you experience on a regular basis.

❑ Mad	❑ Excited	❑ Sad
❑ Annoyed	❑ Happy	❑ Fearful
❑ Frustrated	❑ Ashamed	❑ Joyful
❑ Expectant	❑ Embarrassed	❑ Annoyed
❑ Enraged	❑ Panicked	❑ Peaceful
❑ Hopeful	❑ Motivated	❑ Nervous
❑ Jealous	❑ Worried	❑ Inspired
❑ Loved	❑ Lonely	❑ Ecstatic

- Feelings I attempt to not feel the most _____

_____

- I do this in the following ways _____

_____

_____

- I am most likely to experience positive emotions with _____
  _____

- I am most likely to experience negative emotions with _____
  _____

- I will work on expressing my emotions better to _____
  _____

Tool #11: Increase Socialization

This one seems obvious. But it is the most difficult one for many people with APD. Just about every tool in this chapter will involve being around people. So the more you can do to expose yourself to people, the better. You don't even have to talk to them to start with! Just try to get used to being around them. Even if you don't interact, the exposure will start to increase your comfort level which will benefit you in some of the work you will do later on. Look back to your circles. Who are the people that are closest to you? Where do they hang out? Is it somewhere you could tag along? List five places you *could* go to at least be around other people. Use the following log to help yourself monitor small steps of progress in key areas of your life.

1. _____
2. _____
3. _____
4. _____
5. _____

Tool #12: Avoid Being Hurt

The top priority for people with APD is to keep from getting hurt. It is important to validate that this is not a frivolous desire. Nobody wants to get hurt. However, the avoidant individual fears getting hurt so strongly that this fear drives them to avoid people, fun, and the things they actually want to do in life. Rather than striving to do something, they are striving not to do something. They are playing defense their entire life. Treatment thus, involves impart, helping them shift from defense to offense.

One idea that is important to understand is that avoiding being hurt doesn't have to keep us from achieving our goals. It is possible to pursue the things we want life in ways that minimize the likelihood of getting hurt. So, rather than thinking in "either-or" terms (avoid life or live life), try to think "yes, and…"

Ask yourself the questions:

- What would I enjoy doing? _____
_____
_____

- How can I go about that in the safest way possible? _____
_____
_____

Avoid and Achieve

- Three things I would like to experience in life that I have not been able to so far due to my avoidance are

    1. _____
    2. _____
    3. _____

Now, for each of those items, list the three least intimidating ways you can think of to pursue your goal.

Experiences in Life I Would Like to Have If I Didn't Avoid	Steps I Could Take to Pursue Them with the Least Risk of Getting Hurt
1.	1. 2. 3.
2.	1. 2. 3.
3.	1. 2. 3.

My Reaction _____

_____

_____

Tool #13: Taking Risks

Avoidance actually fuels anxiety. Anxiety is developed and perpetuated by believing something is more threatening than it really is and by minimizing our own ability to cope with that perceived or actual threat. To avoid triggers for anxiety, then, it is common for people to cope by using what are called *safety behaviors*.

Safety behaviors are any behaviors that decrease anxiety in the short term (so that the person feels "safe") but in actuality make the anxiety worse in the long term. In the case of people with APD, these perceived threats typically involve people. If you have APD, you likely have some very specific go-to behaviors you engage in to avoid people. Some people don't go in public at all; others ask friends to do their shopping; some do everything online; and others refuse to listen to voicemails or return calls.

To improve, these behaviors eventually need to be confronted and changed. This involves taking risks that can be quite scary. But you have proven you can do scary things, right?

Us the following tool to identify 1) safety behaviors you engage in with people, 2) goals you listed in the previous tool, and 3) risks that might be involved in accomplishing those goals. Look at the example provided, then complete your own.

Safety Behavior	Goal	Risk
Not answering phone if Suzie calls	Get my degree	1. Talk to Suzie 2. Go with her to school campus

The risk I am willing to take this week

Safety Behavior	Goal	Risk

Tool #14: Untangling the Web of Excuses

You may have heard the expression, "Excuses are like armpits – everybody has a couple, and they stink!" Well, the problem is that people with APD don't just have a couple. They have an entire web of excuses.

You may have noted at the beginning of this chapter that rationalization is one of the common distortions involved. Most people think of rationalization as giving one's self permission to do something harmful. This may be what happens most frequently. But people with APD rationalize in a different way. They give themselves permission to *not* do things that would benefit them. This usually involves avoiding fears, which almost always revolve around other people. Doing what needs to be done to face your fears will come easier if you can untangle some of these webs first.

Use the following format to identify some of the excuses you have woven your web with. The fancy CBT term is *permission-giving beliefs*. Then use the thought log tool to challenge this permission-giving self-talk. Get some help from your therapist, family, or friends if you need to. Come up with a list of reasons why it is not okay to avoid behaviors in whatever area it would benefit you to take risks.

Example: Avoidant Thought Log

Avoidant Thought	Rational Responses
It's ok to NOT _____ (Risk I am avoiding taking) Because _____ (My excuse)	

Tool #15: Face Your Fears

In my *CBT Toolbox* (Riggenbach 2013) I copied with permission part of this tool from Marty Antony (Antony 2018) where he highlighted that in 1999, then-U.S. Surgeon General David Satcher wrote perhaps the most complete review of mental health and treatment ever published. In it he stated that the most important and critical part of treatment for anxiety is "exposure to stimuli"— in other words, facing one's fears. You may have heard the alternative term *exposure*. Exposure is probably the most important strategy for recovery. Unfortunately, it can also be the most difficult, because it requires you to do the things you fear the most. This obviously involves being willing to gradually work to reduce the safety behaviors you identified in Tool #13. It's one thing to tell yourself something isn't as scary as you thought it was; it's another thing to prove it to yourself. Exposure-based strategies are based on the principle that we all get used to things over time.

Although extremely effective when done properly, exposure therapy can otherwise often be harmful, so it is best that you plan this series of exercises with your therapist. As you plan to face your fears, remember one thing: The goal is not to do the exercise without experiencing any anxiety. The goal is to test your belief to see if your fearful perceptions are true. If they aren't true, as you *experience* this over time, your brain learns to process threats differently and your anxiety will decrease. Anxiety typically decreases with gradual exposure over time, and anxiety is the number one obstacle holding people with APD back from doing the things they want to do.

There are many ways to work with exposure, and there are seemingly hundreds of forms out there to help facilitate it. I prefer one used in Marty Antony's *The Anti-Anxiety Handbook*, which I have copied below with permission. Use this tool to track the results of your belief-testing as you face your fears!

Example: Exposure Log

Date	Belief	Pre-test (%)	Test	Result	Post-test (%)
6/13	Bridge will collapse if I go over it	95%	Visualize driving over bridge	Made it safely, bridge didn't collapse	90%
6/15		85%	Watch other cars drive over bridge	55 cars crossed safely in 1 hour, none fell through	80%
6/17		85%	Drove over bridge myself first time	Made it safely, bridge didn't collapse	60%

My Exposure Log

Date	Belief	Pre-test (%)	Test	Result	Post-test (%)

CHAPTER 4: THE DEPENDENT PERSONALITY DISORDER

The Dependent Personality Disorder

Hidden agenda: To be taken care of

Prevalence rates: 1-3% of the general population

Gender distribution: Significantly more common in women than men

Cognitive profile:

- View of self: "I am helpless," "I am incompetent"

- View of others: "Others are competent," "Others are supportive"

- View of world: "The world is overwhelming," "I can only survive with others' help"

Common schemas: Dependence, enmeshment, subjugation

Common cognitive distortions: Discounting the positive, fortune telling, mind reading, "should" statements (directed toward selves)

Overdeveloped traits: Help-seeking, clinging behaviors

Underdeveloped traits: Self-sufficiency, independence

Whom they date/marry: Narcissists, other controlling or domineering people

Where they work: Low-level military, secretarial positions, assembly lines

Other Random Nuggets:

Continuum

Mild	Moderate	Severe
Mildly submissive Constantly lonely if not involved Functions well with good "fits" in relationships and work	Difficulty spending time alone Must be romantically involved Must have "hand held" constantly	Helpless to live life Requires others to significantly care for them

Tool #1: Trait Checklist

Individuals that suffer from the characteristics of dependent personality disorder (DPD) have a number of commonalities. Whether you or a loved one has this full blown condition, or some of the traits of it, survey the following checklist. The more of these you checkmark, the more likely it is this pattern of behavior is causing some problems occupationally, relationally, or socially.

- ❏ Feels a constant need to be in a relationship

- ❏ When one relationship ends, finds new caretaker to take over major responsibilities in life

- ❏ Has difficulty disagreeing with others

- ❏ Needs frequent reassurance

- ❏ Needs more "quality time" with partner than most

- ❏ Can't be alone

- ❏ Has difficulty initiating tasks or projects

- ❏ Asks for help more often than others without trying things on own

- ❏ Needs significantly more physical touch than others

- ❏ Has difficulty making decisions on their own

- ❏ Has few if any hobbies to do on own which are not tied to significant other

- ❏ Has few friends outside of current "caretaker"

Tool #2: Expressions of Concern

All people have what are often called "blind spots": qualities we don't see in ourselves as well as others see in us. Because of the ego-syntonic nature of PDs, this phenomenon is particularly challenging for these people. What this means practically is that things that pose problems for friends and family members are often not are considered problematic by the individual with the condition. Concerns expressed by friends and family may have validity to them, but due to poor insight, the PD individual generally has difficulty seeing how certain behaviors impact themselves or others negatively. However, not all concerns friends and family express have validity. So, one of the tough but vital steps for recovery is sorting through these "complaints" to determine which ones have validity and which ones do not. People with dependent traits usually value others opinions significantly, so this exercise can be motivating for this population.

Use the following tool to identify *who* has expressed concern, *what* the exact concerns are, and *why* they see them as potentially hurtful. Look at the example, then complete your own and answer the questions that follow.

Example:

Person Expressing Concern	Action Causing Concern	Reason for Concern
1. Aunt 2. Mom 3. Aunt (same one)	1. Spends too much time with mother and not people my age 2. Ignoring all my friends after I got a boyfriend 3. I am 27 and have never had a job	1. Worry that I will never "get a life" 2. Boys will come and go but friends are supposed to be for a lifetime. 3. Worry that when my mom dies I won't be able to take care of myself

Questions:

- Who are three people I trust to "shoot straight" with me, by whom I can run these concerns to get their opinion?

    1. Aunt

    2. Cousin

    3. Boyfriend

- With which concerns can I at least see where the person is coming from?

    Too much time with boyfriend and not as much time with friends—I am going to marry him

- Which concerns can I see the MOST validity in?

    I do want to be able to take care of myself

- I am willing to take the following steps to change one of the concerns:

    1. Look online for a job

    2. Call Judi

    3. ?

My Expressions of Concern

Person Expressing Concern	Action Causing Concern	Reason for Concern
1.	1.	1.
2.	2.	2.
3.	3.	3.
4.	4.	4.
5.	5.	5.

Questions:

- Who are three people I trust to "shoot straight" with me, by whom I can run these concerns to get their opinion?

    1. _____

    2. _____

    3. _____

- With which concerns can I at least see where the person is coming from? _____
  _____
  _____

- Which concerns can I see the most validity in? _____
  _____
  _____

- I am willing to take the following steps to change one of the concerns
  1. _____
  2. _____
  3. _____

Tool #3: Pros and Cons

This tool helps you evaluate the potential pros and cons of your dependent behaviors. It is called a *four box pros and cons*. Sometimes it can be beneficial to look at not only the advantages and disadvantages of maintaining certain behaviors but also the advantages and disadvantages of changing them. After listing the pros and cons of each, it can be even more helpful to rate, on a scale of 0-10, how important each item is. Consider the example that is provided. Then complete one on your own!

Example: Pros and Cons of Perfectionistic Behavior

Pros of Remaining Dependent	Pros of Becoming More Independent
He takes care of me (7)	Would have a job (6)
I don't have to work (7)	Would have my own money (10)
I don't have to pay the bills or stuff like that (8)	Could see my old friends once in a while (5)
Cons of Remaining Dependent	**Cons of Becoming More Independent**
Only get small allowance to spend (8)	My husband would be mad at me (10)
Don't have anything that is my own (4)	I'd have to work (8)
My friend Claire is mad I never go out with her (9)	I'm scared I wouldn't know what to do (5)
	Life would be harder (6)

Results:

__22__ Reasons to remain dependent

__21__ Reasons to not remain dependent

__21__ Reasons to become more independent

__29__ Reasons to not become more independent

My Conclusions: I could have a lot more things I want and a lot more fun in life if I weren't scared 1) that I couldn't do it and 2) of what my husband might do.

My Commitments: I will go to coffee with Claire and let her tell me about her job.

Analysis: This woman in her late 30s is just starting to realize she is missing out in life, mainly thanks to pressure from her friend Claire. She can "sniff" a more enriched life, but is still petrified by responsibility and how her husband might react to her changing. Her result numbers are strikingly even, so we have some motivating factors to work with. She is resistant to take too many steps, but she has committed to one. That is a start.

My Pros and Cons of Dependent Behavior

Pros of Remaining Dependent	Pros of Becoming More Independent
Cons of Remaining Dependent	**Cons of Becoming More Independent**

Results:

_____ Reasons to remain dependent

_____ Reasons to not remain dependent

_____ Reasons to become more independent

_____ Reasons to not become more independent

My Conclusions _____

_____

_____

_____

My Commitment _____

_____

_____

_____

_____

Tool #4: Identify Behavioral Targets

Dependent traits manifest differently in different people. Some behaviors include difficulty being assertive with people in life, and becoming overly reliant on one person (putting all of one's "emotional eggs" in one basket, constant phone calls and , texts, demands for time, other needy behaviors). Some have difficulty leaving unhealthy or abusive relationships. Some have a very difficult time being alone and, if a relationship ends, will immediately take the first thing that comes along, so to speak, to not be alone. Some find others in life to be with who will take on that responsibility on their behalf. If they are not in a romantic relationship, it is common that they still live with parents or other family members. They almost always ask for help rather than attempt a task on their own. They are often experienced as "draining" or needy by significant others.

Use this tool to identify some of your dependent behaviors that you or others have noticed to target in treatment. Feel free to use any of the above behaviors that fit you, or list some of your own.

- **Behaviors related to my dependence traits that I or someone else identified which I am willing to target to improve my situation**

    1. _____
    2. _____
    3. _____
    4. _____
    5. _____

Tool #5: Intimacy Circles

Intimacy is a scary word for a lot of people. If the sound of it makes you cringe, this exercise is definitely for you—and even if it doesn't, this exercise likely will still benefit you. It will benefit almost everyone in some way. Why? Because almost everyone could benefit from improving at least one interpersonal relationship in their life. Some people's lives could be enriched with more friends. Others need to learn to set boundaries with someone in their life. A lot of people have "trust issues." Yet others would be happier in life if they learned to pick healthier people to date or form friendships with; toxic people have a way of draining people of their energy and joy. A certain percentage of the population would be much less prone to mood swings if they could be okay alone. Some would find more fulfillment in life if they could share more with people in their lives; others would not be hurt as often if they learned to share less with those in their life. A lot of people walk around with their "walls" up. Some have difficulty expressing feelings. Some have been accused of being too "needy." Others have difficulty asking for help.

You may have heard intimacy defined as "Into-Me-See"—the degree to which we let people see into us, and vice versa. A lot of my clients have found this "play on words" to be a helpful way to remember its definition and connotations.

Use the following tool to evaluate the relationships in your life. Use the percentage signs to help you decide which people to put in which circles. No other person goes in the ME circle (though some people choose to put God here). This is for you alone. People who belong in circle #1 are those with whom you would feel comfortable sharing ANY problem in life, no matter how personal (a sexual problem, something related to an abusive situation, a salary issue, etc.). People in circle #2 are those in your life with whom there may be a personal issue or two (like the ones mentioned above) that you would not share, but you would be comfortable sharing ALMOST anything (roughly 75%) about your life. People in circle #3 may get about half of your personal stuff, but the other half you probably would not trust them with. People in circle #4 would be your very casual relationships. Maybe they know whether you are married or where you work or something of that nature, but you don't share very much with them (roughly 25%). And people in circle #5 get nothing. For some people, these are individuals whom they have just met, so they could be candidates to move closer in as they get to know them. Or, these are people who at one point in life were closer in, but they have done something to violate trust, so they have had to be moved out one or more rings.

If you have dependent traits, you are likely a "people person." If so, this activity may be fun for you. Although it can be enjoyable to look at and think about relationships, making beneficial changes can be quite scary—if this is you, remember your tendencies to over-rely on others, specifically one significant caretaker figure in your life. Consider the person in your life on whom it would be beneficial to decrease your dependency and the person(s) in your life with whom it might benefit you to spend more time, as well as what unhealthy relationships you may have had difficulty letting go of up until now.

Keep these ideas in mind as you consider who truly belongs where as you complete your circles. Your first task is to think about all the people in your life and where they go in your circles. Then consider the questions that follow. Whether you are able to use this tool to improve your own relationships or if you choose to follow up with some coaching to get assistance with someone in your life, I hope you find it to be a useful tool.

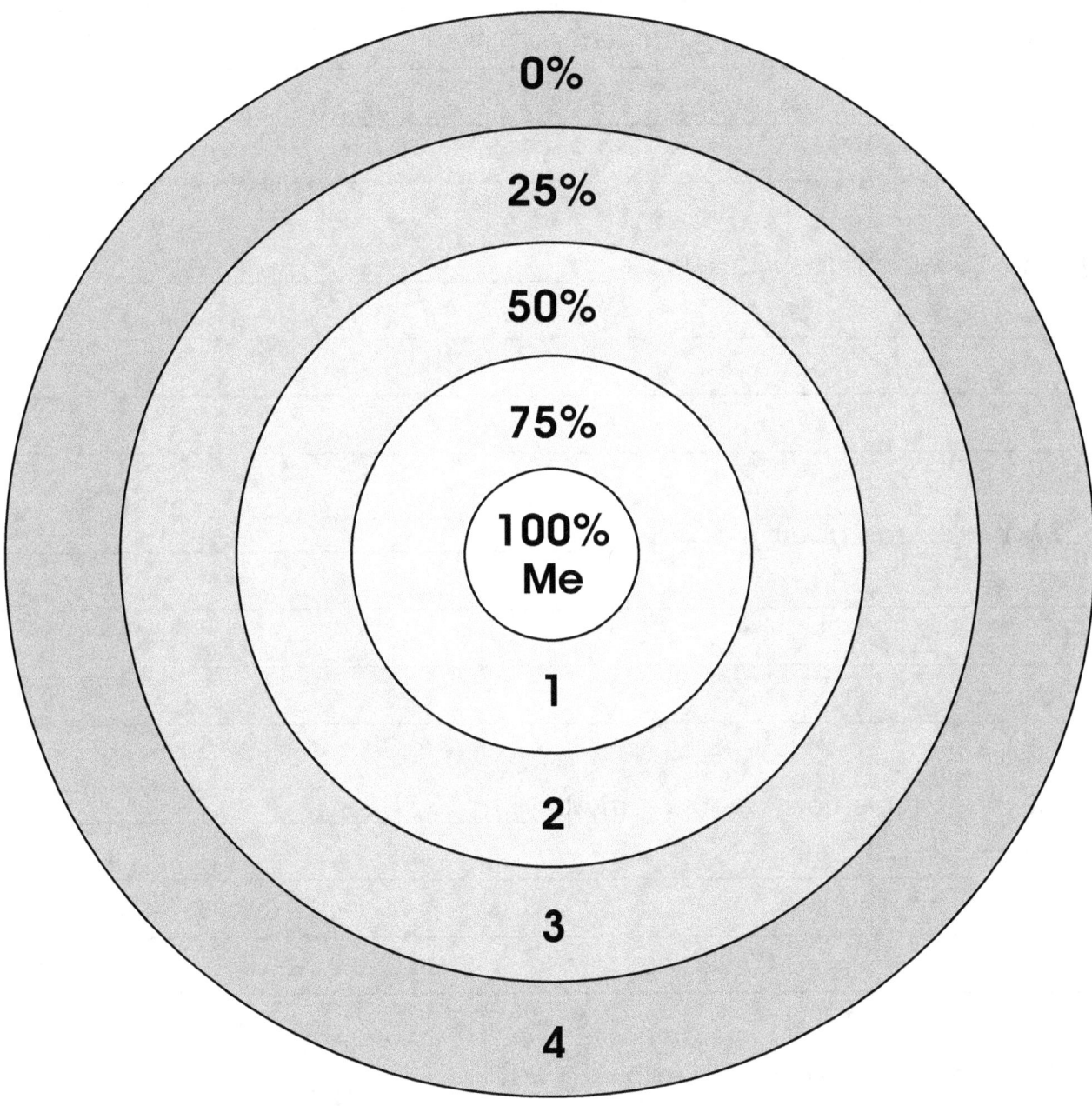

Intimacy Circles Follow-Up Starter Questions

- General observations about my circles _____
  _____
  _____
  _____

- What I like most about my circles _____
  _____
  _____
  _____

- What I like least about my circles _____
  _____
  _____
  _____

- The most problematic people in my life _____
  _____
  _____
  _____

- They are problematic in the following ways _____
  _____
  _____
  _____

- People in my life whose opinions I actually care about and on a scale of 0-10 how much I care what they think _____

_____

_____

_____

- People in my life whose opinions I don't care about _____

_____

_____

- People in my life whom I have hurt/violated/taken advantage of _____

_____

_____

_____

- People in my life who have moved themselves out in my circles due to my behavior

_____

_____

_____

- I could improve my circles if I were willing to keep the following rules (which I have not previously been willing to keep) _____

_____

_____

_____

- One step I will take TODAY to improve my relationship circles _____

_____

_____

Tool #6: Identify and Restructure Automatic Thoughts

A staple component of treatment for any psychological condition is recognizing the thought processes that are driving the problem behaviors and maintaining the symptoms. In colloquial language, you may hear this referred to as "self-talk." To speak in the terms of the Mark Twain quote in Chapter 1 ("If all you have is a hammer, everything looks like a nail"): This is the "hammer." While treatment of personality disorders requires more tools than just a hammer, the hammer is still a useful tool to have in your toolbox.

Some people develop an awareness of their thoughts and get better at noticing them, but do nothing to change them. For example, if we recognize that we are overweight, but do nothing to change our diets or exercise levels, we will stay overweight. In the same way, if we recognize thoughts that are driving problem behavior but do nothing to change them, our symptoms are likely to remain.

So, one cognitive tool you can use is what is called *challenging distorted thoughts* when you recognize them. Refer to the beginning of this chapter for some distorted thoughts common in avoidant personality disorder. *"Challenging,"* in this case, basically means arguing with the specific content of the thoughts. There are a number of techniques that can be used for doing this, including looking at evidence, seeking input from others, researching the facts, considering past or possible future results, or good old-fashioned logic, just to name a few.

The following tool asks you to identify specific dependent thoughts that enter your mind, challenge them in some way, and if you want to, rate your challenge on a scale of 0-10 to indicate how meaningful the challenge is. Take a look at the example, and then do one on your own. This may be a tool that you benefit from using on an ongoing basis.

Example: Thought Log

Distorted Thought	Rational Responses
If I argue with him again he might leave me. Since I could never make it on my own, it's best that I just do what he asks	We have argued before and he has never left I was lonely, but I made it by myself before I met him If I do what he asks every time, I never get to do things that I enjoy I am capable of doing things on my own—my needs are important too

Dependent Thought Log

Dependent Thought	Rational Responses

Tool #7: Historical Experiences Worksheet

Dependent personality disorder may be the least researched condition in this category of diagnoses. It also may have the lowest genetic concordance rate. While it is believed that it is largely a product of environment, exact experiences have not been considered in depth. Peruse the following historical experiences that seem to be common in people with this disorder. Put an "X" beside factors that were a part of your experiences from a young age.

- ❑ Had one or more overprotective parent(s)
- ❑ Had multiple siblings
- ❑ Parents never taught children basic skills
- ❑ Parents never taught decision making
- ❑ Parents failed to foster taking responsibility
- ❑ Experienced a major loss early in life
- ❑ Background did not encourage development of hobbies or interests
- ❑ Independence was not valued

- Describe how the experiences checked above apply specifically to you and the impact you believe they continue to have in your life today

_____
_____
_____
_____
_____
_____
_____
_____
_____
_____
_____

Tool #8: Belief Identification

As has been discussed, all behaviors are a product of beliefs. Beliefs drive behavior. Due to the compelling nature of beliefs in individuals with PDs, these deeper-level beliefs often have to be modified to help create lasting change. As noted at the beginning of this chapter, common beliefs in people with DPD include approval seeking, social isolation, and emotional inhibition, among others. Review their definitions if you don't have them fresh in your mind. Get with your therapist. Include friends and family who are willing to give you feedback. Identify one or two beliefs that you believe drive your target behaviors to work on in treatment. Write them inside Judy Beck's "Pac-Man" visual aid (which was explained in the introduction)..

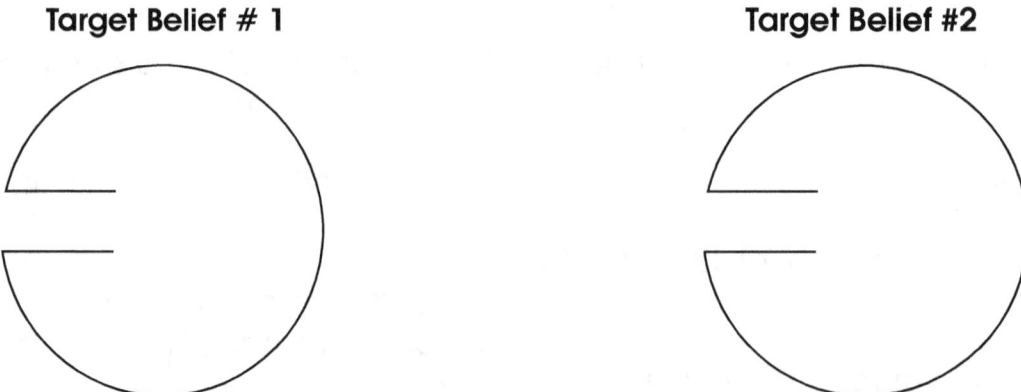

Beliefs always come in pairs. For every maladaptive (or unhealthy) belief we possess, we also possess an alternate, adaptive (or healthy) belief. For instance, even though an individual may have the belief, "I must isolate myself because I am a social outcast," they also have the belief, however faint, "I can fit in."

I have given you the "pushing buttons" language, the "Pac-Man" visual, and the "filters" imagery. Here is another representation which I hope helps illustrate the point: We could think of beliefs as lenses. For people who wear glasses, this visual probably comes fairly intuitively. Healthier individuals are able to engage in more balanced information processing. Figuratively speaking they are able to see out of both the left and the right "lenses" equally. This is the goal of belief modification work: balanced information processing. In other words, to be able to see both sides objectively and to be able to recognize when they fail or make mistakes, so they can learn from them; and also to be able to acknowledge when they succeed and be able to take a compliment. Although nobody is perfect and everyone has their biases, healthier people's lenses are closer to the 50/50 range (50% failure/50% success). Before treatment, people with PDs, due to their more compelling beliefs, often start with numbers such as 99%/1%. *Intentional and sustained effort* is required to create a healthier belief balance.

So, now that you have identified your unhealthy beliefs driving your target behaviors, identify in your own words what you would call the opposite, healthy belief. Write it in the opposite belief structure that the "triangle" could fit into.

After you have identified your one or two healthy and unhealthy beliefs, ask yourself: "What percentage of the time do I believe the unhealthy belief? What percentage of the time do I believe the healthy belief?" Write your numbers in the line next to each belief (they should total 100%). Then you are ready to move on to Tool #9!

See the example first, and then do one on your own!

Example: Belief Identification

Target Belief #1	Healthy Belief #1
"Need others to survive"	"Can be self-sufficient"
95% Strength	5% Strength

Target Belief #2	Healthy Belief #2
Strength	Strength

My Beliefs

Target Belief #1	Healthy Belief #1
_____ Strength	_____ Strength
Target Belief #2	**Healthy Belief #2**
_____ Strength	_____ Strength

Tool #9: Evidence Logs

Here is where the hard work begins! This is a tool you will use throughout your treatment, regardless of what other tools you may be using and at what stage of treatment you may be at. This is the tough, tough work of gradually working to develop your healthy belief. How do we change beliefs, anyway? It's a difficult process, no doubt. What we need to do is to *reexamine historical evidence, get better at noticing current evidence* **and** *intentionality initiate ongoing experiences around which to create new evidence.*

Think of any belief that you have changed over time in any area of your life. Maybe you used to not believe in God and now you do. Perhaps you used to not believe in global warming and now you do. Maybe you used to believe in life on other planets and now you don't. For example, I have a client who is a marine biology major in college – his chief interest is in Megalodon sharks, which he was initially convinced were not extinct. After a lot of scientific research, he now no longer believes that. Did you used to hold more conservative political beliefs, and your beliefs are now more progressive? You get the gist. You can use a belief that you have changed in any area of life to illustrate this process. How do

beliefs change? By examining the evidence created by experience and the meaning that we assign to it.

Take a belief many people once held. (WARNING! UPCOMING CONTENT NOT APPROPRIATE FOR KIDS!) Santa Claus is not real. If you believed in his existence when you were six years old, what was the "evidence" that supported your belief? He brought presents. They said "from Santa" on the wrapping. He drank the milk that was set out for him. He knew what presents were desired from the letters that was sent to him at the North Pole. The local weather even tracks him on the Doppler radar!

Over time, most people reexamine the pieces of evidence and assign new meaning to them. By doing so, they change their belief.

But they have to *experience* new evidence.

Some children recognize Papa beneath the Santa suit and false white beard. Some children stay up all night and sneak downstairs to catch a parent putting presents under the tree. Some children are observant enough to notice that "Santa" has Mommy's identical hand writing or wrapping paper. The child who does *not* go out of their way to look for these things holds onto the old, false belief much longer because they are not looking for evidence to the contrary. In fact, when I myself was becoming suspicious but desperately wanted to believe that he was real as a child, I began actively searching out confirmation of his existence.

In the same way, for any of us to change our beliefs, we must be *willing* to examine evidence fairly. We are naturally (consciously or unconsciously) looking for evidence to support our existing belief. But we must be equally willing to consider evidence to the contrary as well. This is what the evidence logs do: they provide a tool to facilitate *purposefully looking for evidence* to support the new belief you are attempting to construct. If your current unhealthy belief is that you are a failure, then you are purposefully looking for evidence that you can succeed. For some cognitive behavioral therapy (CBT) exercises, we will ask people to log evidence on *both* sides. But because people with PDs have such deeply engrained beliefs, their natural tendency will be to see only evidence that supports the current belief. So, for the purpose of this exercise, it is important to use the right column only to log evidence that supports the belief. The left column will remain blank.

As you record the evidence, think about how it felt to have that experience. As you do, ask yourself: *In this moment* how much do I believe _____ and how much do I believe _____?
　　　　　　　　　　　　　　　　　　　(unhealthy belief)　　　　　　　　　　　　　　　　　　　　(healthy belief)

Remember, you will inherently *not notice* evidence that will be helpful because your filter is directing you away from it, so be vigilant. Also, when you log evidence for a healthy belief, you will get that little voice in your head that says, "but… it doesn't count because of this or that." Go ahead and record the evidence anyway even if you have trouble believing it at the time.

Log the believability rating as you record each piece of evidence. Note that these numbers will go up

and down, because beliefs fluctuate. But over time, watch your unhealthy numbers generally trend down and your healthy numbers trend up. The more they change, the more balanced your lenses will be come and you will get your "buttons pushed" less frequently!

Look at the example below. Then begin completing your own evidence log, working on one belief at a time. When you have more than one icebergs to conquer, the more effort you put into chiseling one at a time, the more progress you will make.

Example: Evidence Log

Unhealthy Belief: 95%   Healthy Belief: 5%

Date	"Need others to survive"	% Belief	"Can be self-sufficient"	% Belief
4/12		75%	Paid the bills myself this month	25%
4/13		80%	Made my own doctor appointment and got there myself	20%
4/14		55%	Made it on my own when my mom went out of town for three days	45%
4/16		70%	Did my own laundry	30%

Conclusions: I can do things I just never even tried to do before.

My Evidence Log

Unhealthy Belief: **Healthy Belief:**

Date		% Belief		% Belief

Conclusions _____

_____

Tool #10: Getting Taken Care Of

At their core, the person with DPD just wants to be sure they are taken care of. All humans have basic needs that have to be met, so it is understandable that someone can experience discomfort if they believe they are not going to get these needs fulfilled. One problem with the individual with DPD is that often times they have never developed some of the basic skills necessary to take care of themselves and their lives. While skill building is a vital component of getting better, until those tools have been added to the toolbox, it is likely necessary to rely on others.

As was alluded to in Tool #5 (the "circles" exercise), a common issue in this population is putting all of one's emotional eggs in one basket. Often times this "basket" is a parent; frequently it is a spouse; it could be anybody. But there are clear down sides to this "dumping" strategy: the person who is completely and whole-heartedly relied on could leave, die, or become unavailable when needed; or, if conflict arises between the two, the situation is extremely uncomfortable for the person with DPD. Another common by product of this dependent relationship is that the relied-upon person can easily become burned out. So, without realizing it, the DPD individual may inadvertently push them away and create the very circumstances they fear the most.

It can be helpful, therefore, to "spread out your neediness," so to speak, as you are working to decrease it. The following tool will ask you to identify three people you can go to in your life to help you in different areas. For instance, you may have one person you go to when you are lonely, another to help with finances, a third to help with household projects and maintenance, and somebody completely different to go out and have fun with. Use the following tool to identify your support people as well as areas that you will go to them for help.

Getting Your Needs Met Tool

Support Person #1 _____

Support Person #2 _____

Support Person #3 _____

Tool #11: Gaining Independence

When we don't have the ability to meet our own needs, it is great to have people who can help us do so. Hopefully you were able to identify some of those people and how to "spread out your neediness" so as not to be so reliant on one person in the previous section. The next crucial step is ***building some skills*** so that you gain the ability to meet some of your own needs. Some people have skill deficits in only one or two major areas, whereas others have deficits in multiple areas. This tool is designed to help you think about some of those areas and assess to what degree skills might need to be developed in each.

What I CAN Do	What I CAN'T Do
What I CAN Do	**What I CAN'T Do**
What I CAN Do	**What I CAN'T Do**
What I CAN Do	**What I CAN'T Do**
What I CAN Do	**What I CAN'T Do**

Conclusions _____

_____

_____

Commitment Steps _____

_____

_____

Tool #12: Positive Self-Image

The central issue at the core of DPD is negative beliefs about self, or what clients may call "self-esteem." Self-esteem doesn't appear out of thin air. We can't just repeat positive affirmations that deep down we don't believe all day long and then expect self-esteem to appear overnight. Maybe you remember the line from *What About Bob?* in which Bill Murray's character, Bob Wiley, states, "I feel good, I feel great, I feel wonderful," over and over and over. Yet, no matter how many times he recited those words, it was obvious that repetition alone didn't help him believe them.

Core beliefs about self, i.e., "self-image," grow slowly over time as we do things that we consider worthwhile or as we gain attributes that we value **and** are able to give ourselves credit. Most people with low self-esteem don't have this image of themselves because they don't have admirable qualities; they have this image because they are not able to give themselves credit for the positive traits they have.

If you don't have positive qualities (highly unlikely, as everyone has positive qualities) or skillfulness in certain areas, you need to continue to work the previous tool (#11) to develop them. After that, the next step is to identify the particular positive qualities, attributes, and skills that we have so that we can start working to give ourselves credit for them. It does little good to build the skills if we can't *see* the skills.

The following tool will help you do just that. While these may be hard to see in yourself at first, make your best effort to list one positive quality you have demonstrated, even if only at times, for each letter of the alphabet. Seek help from friends or family if you have difficulty. If you find yourself hesitating on a particular quality or skill, even if you don't 100% believe you have it, force yourself to write it down anyway. As has been discussed, believability increases over time. After all, if you already believed these things, you wouldn't have to do this exercise and likely wouldn't be working this book!

Alphabet Attributes Tool: Positive Qualities from A-Z!

A _____

B _____

C _____

D _____

E _____

F _____

G _____

H _____

I _____

J _____

K _____

L _____

M _____

N _____

O _____

P _____

Q _____

R _____

S _____

T _____

U _____

V _____

W _____

X _____

Y _____

Z _____

My Reaction _____
_____
_____
_____

Tool #13: Expanding Identity

Great job if you have completed the previous two tools! Once you have *built the skills* the next step is to start to incorporate these into your identity. We have a lot of skills or qualities we don't identify with. I always joke that I brush my teeth every day, but I never introduce myself to someone new by saying, "Nice to meet you—I am Jeff the toothbrusher." So just because we do something habitually doesn't mean it is important enough to incorporate into the components of our beliefs about ourselves.

Now lets explore this a bit further. Think about the attributes identified above and consider which of them are more important *TO YOU*. This is an important concept, because different people value different things.

For instance, many people value their cultural heritage. They may study their roots, examine the family genealogy, and perform customs even today that were important to their culture historically. Some people gain a deep sense of connection and satisfaction from this.

However, others, such as myself, couldn't care less about this pursuit. Let me tell a personal anecdote: Recently I received a strange email from "Jeff Riggenbach" in my inbox. I do email myself at times, but this one was from another Jeff Riggenbach who lives in California who happened to be doing some research on genealogy. He asked me if I was from the Dutch Riggenbachs or the German Riggenbachs and if I knew this family or that family. He actually had a list of over fifty questions for me! This subject was obviously important to him. Unfortunately, I think I knew the answer to about three of his questions.

All this is to say, a quality or value has to be important to *you*, or else it will not impact your beliefs about yourself, the quality of your relationships, or your moods in day-to-day situations.

For some, identity is a little puzzling. Finding yours starts with answering the question, "How do I define myself?" Identity can be found in religious beliefs, personal strengths, occupations, hobbies, friends, causes we feel strongly about, gender, age, and our relationships to others, to name just a few. You have probably heard the expression, "wearing a lot of hats." Consider for a few minutes the "hats" you wear. In developing identity, it can be helpful to think in terms of ***I am*** (characteristics or qualities identified in Tool #12), ***I have*** (possessions or relationships that aren't inherently part of us, but that are important to us), ***I can*** (skills or capabilities explored in Tool #11), and ***I like*** (personal preferences or hobbies). Look over the example, and then spend a few minutes considering how you might answer these questions. Your answers will provide you a valuable window into which to peek to help slowly develop your identity.

Example:

- I am ... caring, loving, sensitive

- I have ... a loving family

- I can ... knit/play golf

- I like ... cooking

Now, in your own words:

- I am _____

- I have _____

- I can _____

- I like _____

Under each hat in the illustration on the next page, write one of the ways you currently define yourself or of the ways that you may like to see yourself in the future. For instance, one client's "hats" included being a *niece, a sister, a friend, a Christian, a stamp collector, a chef, a secretary, and a movie goer.*

The Hats Tool

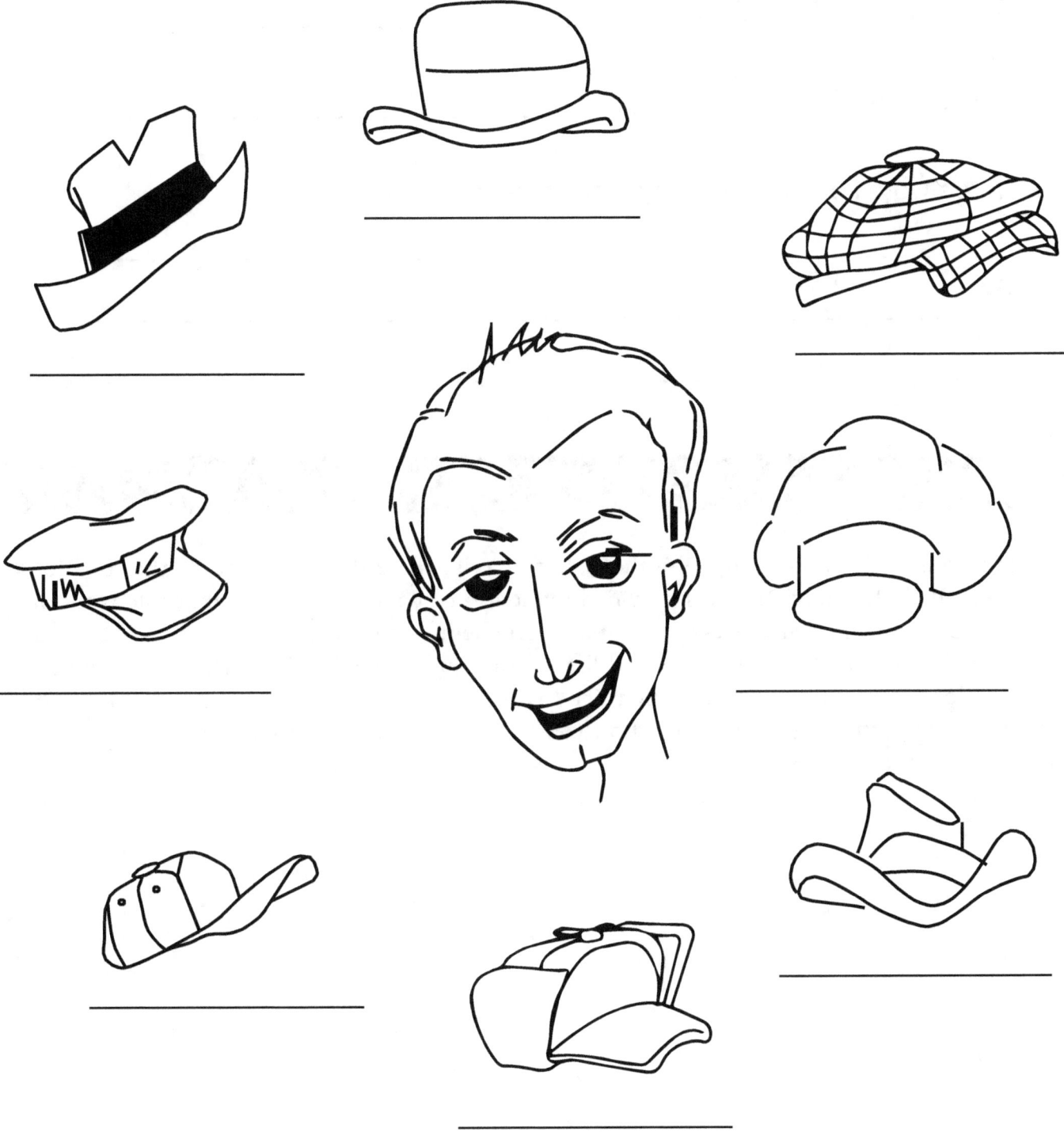

Adapted from Velasquez, Maurer, Crouch, and DiClemente, 2001

Chapter 4: The Dependent Personality Disorder

Strengthening My Identity

- The "hat" I most identify with _____

- The one I least identify with _____

- Three ways I can develop my identity as a
    1. _____
    2. _____
    3. _____

Tool #14: Get a Life!

The title of this tool is a bit tongue-in-cheek, but here is where the rubber meets the road for you if you have DPD. The previous tools provided foundational concepts that some people work on for years. Those fundamentals are necessary but not overly helpful unless one actually goes out and starts living life differently. A diverse and fulfilled life usually eludes people with DPD due to not having the foundational necessities or not putting them to use. Here is where you get to put them to use. Use this tool as an opportunity to think about how you can create a more enjoyable and contented life that is not tied to the status of one relationship.

Communication Style	Negative Results

Tool #15: Becoming Assertive

Now that you are living life and interacting with people, you may be experiencing one particular struggle that almost everyone with even dependent traits undergoes: not getting run over or taken advantage of. Standing up for oneself is a challenge if you don't believe you are worth standing up for or if you don't have the skills to stand up for yourself—even if you believe you don't deserve to be taken advantage of. Hopefully your healthy beliefs about yourself are gradually being strengthened, so this tool is devoted to teaching you some basic assertiveness skills.

Assertiveness in communication with other people has been taught in seemingly a thousand ways. Here is one popular way of characterizing unhealthy communication styles:

1. Passive

2. Aggressive

3. Passive-Aggressive

The abbreviated version of this categorization is that passive individuals have difficulty standing up for themselves; aggressive people stand up for themselves in a way that runs over other people, and passive-aggressive people don't stand up to you to your face, but will get you back in some way later. Passive people don't tell you (ever) that they are upset with you; aggressive people may even get verbally or physically violent to tell you they are upset with you; and passive-aggressive people will not tell you to your face, but will gossip behind your back or slit your tires the next day.

People with dependent traits tend to fall in the "passive" category. Use the following tool to identify your style.

- I would describe my communication style as _____
  _____
  _____

- As a result of my style, I have experienced/am experiencing the following negative results _____
  _____
  _____

- One change I need to make in the way I communicate _____
  _____
  _____

- One person in my life I will try this week to be more assertive with _____
  _____
  _____

The Role of *I*-Statements in Assertive communication

An *I*-statement can be defined as communication of thoughts or feelings beginning with the word "I." Even if in a given argument you are 100% right and the other person is 100% wrong (which is rarely the case), using the word "you" at the beginning of a statement often puts the other person on the defensive. Arguments often escalate not because we are "wrong" or have an invalid or inferior point of view, but because of how we communicate that point of view. Although it is easy to disagree about interpretation of facts, it is hard to argue (although some will try) with how someone feels. The following formula can be used to reframe your thoughts into *I*-statements:

1. What is the problem behavior?

2. Why didn't I like it? Or, how did I feel when it happened?

3. What would I like the other person to do instead next time?

Example: I felt unloved when you gave Tommy and Sarah gifts at the end of the get-together and I was the only sibling without something to remember the trip by. If I had known you had something for me that I would get when we got home, I wouldn't have felt so bad the whole flight back. Would you mind telling me next time?

Although people are certainly responsible for their various behaviors, blaming them is rarely helpful. Nobody thrives in an atmosphere of blame. The other side of the coin is obviously not standing up for yourself at all. If we can't stand up for ourselves we will never get what we want.

The most helpful approach, then, is to assertively communicate what you see the problem to be (without labeling or name-calling) and shifting quickly to an action request – that is, describing what you would like the other person to do.

- What are some problem behaviors in relationships I am in? _____
_____
_____

- What would be an assertive way to communicate those problem behaviors to them (using an *I*-statement)? _____
_____
_____

- This week, I will practice assertive communication with _____

CHAPTER 5: THE HISTRIONIC PERSONALITY DISORDER

The Histrionic Personality Disorder

Hidden agenda: To be noticed (most often by the opposite sex specifically)

Prevalence rates: 2-3% of the general population

Gender distribution: Significantly more commonly diagnosed in women than men

Cognitive profile:

- View of self: "I am beautiful/glamourous"

- View of others: "Others can be seduced"

- View of world: "The world is my stage"

Common schemas: Defectiveness, approval seeking, emotional inhibition (overcompensating style), insufficient self-control

Common cognitive distortions: Personalization, mind reading, magnification, emotional reasoning

Overdeveloped traits: Expressiveness, exhibitionism

Underdeveloped traits: Self-control, reflectiveness

Whom they date/marry: OCPDs, other "stable" and "controlled" people

Where they work: Theatre, fashion, charismatic pastors

Other Random Nuggets: Highest dropout rate of any personality disorder

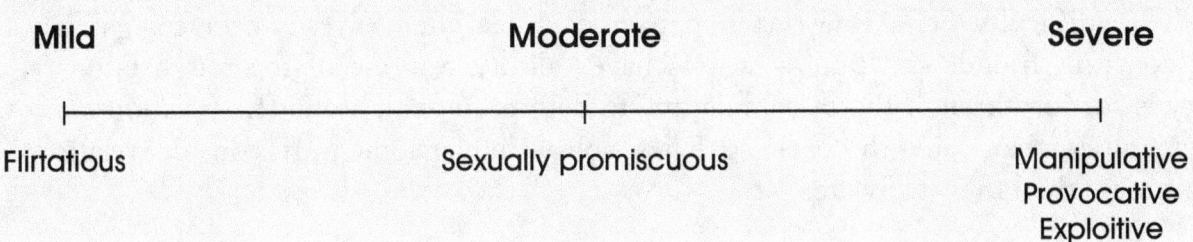

Tool #1: Trait Checklist

Individuals that suffer from the characteristics of histrionic personality disorder (HPD) have a number of commonalities. Whether you are a loved one has this full blown condition, or some of the traits of it, survey the following checklist. The more of these you check yes to, the more likely it is this pattern of behavior is causing some problems occupationally, relationally, or socially.

- ❏ Needs to be the center of attention at all times in public
- ❏ Flirtatious and sexually seductive or provocative behaviors
- ❏ Complains of being "sick" in some way often
- ❏ Vivid expressions
- ❏ Frequent, shallow mood swings
- ❏ Physical attraction is the most valuable quality (in themselves and others)
- ❏ Uses physical appearance to get others' attention
- ❏ Can talk seemingly forever and say nothing of substance
- ❏ Is known as a "drama queen" for excessive emotionality and impulsivity
- ❏ Views relationships consistently as more intimate than the other person does

Tool #2: Expressions of Concern

All people have what are often called "blind spots": qualities we don't see in ourselves as well as others see in us. Because of the ego-syntonic nature of PDs, this phenomenon is particularly challenging for these people. What this means practically is that things that pose problems for friends and family members are often not are considered problematic by the individual with the condition. Concerns expressed by friends and family may have validity to them, but due to poor insight, the PD individual generally has difficulty seeing how certain behaviors impact themselves or others negatively. However, not all concerns friends and family express have validity. So, one of the tough but vital steps for recovery is sorting through these "complaints" to determine which ones have validity and which do not. Remember when doing this exercise that people with histrionic traits consider relationships to be more intimate than they really are.

Use the following tool to identify *who* has expressed concern, *what* the exact concerns are, and *why* they see them as potentially hurtful. Look at the example, then complete your own and answer the questions that follow.

Example:

Person Expressing Concern	Action Causing Concern	Reason for Concern
1. Katy (friend from church)	1. Having affair with manager	1. Negatively affect self-esteem/self-image
2. Sara (cousin)	2. Affair with manager; multiple plastic surgeries	2. Hurt reputation/career trajectory; not healthy
3. Father	3. Drinking alcohol	3. Alcoholic, health concerns

Questions:

- Who are three people I trust to "shoot straight" with me, by whom I can run these concerns to get their opinion?

    1. Sara

    2. Katy

    3. ?

- With which concerns can I at least see where the "complainer" is coming from?

    So far, the affair has helped my career

- I am willing to take the following steps to change one of the concerns
    1. Start going to AA meetings
    2. Start going with Katy to her accountability partner meetings
    3. ?

My Expressions of Concern

Person Expressing Concern	Action Causing Concern	Reason for Concern
1.	1.	1.
2.	2.	2.
3.	3.	3.
4.	4.	4.
5.	5.	5.

Questions:

- With which concerns can I at least see where the person is coming from? _____
  _____
  _____

- Which concerns can I see the most validity in? _____
  _____
  _____

- I am willing to take the following steps to change one of the concerns
    1. _____
    2. _____
    3. _____

Tool #3: Pros and Cons

This tool helps you evaluate the potential pros and cons of your histrionic behaviors. It is called a *four box pros and cons*. Sometimes it can be beneficial to look at not only the advantages and disadvantages of maintaining certain behaviors but also the advantages and disadvantages of changing them. After listing the pros and cons of each, it can be even more helpful to rate, on a scale of 0-10, how important each item is. Consider the example that is provided. Then complete one on your own!

Example: Pros and Cons of Attention-Seeking Behavior

Pros of Remaining Attention-Seeking	Pros of Decreasing Attention Seeking
I feel good when guys talk to me (6)	I might respect myself more (6)
It has helped me "climb the ladder" (5)	I might have different friends (9)
Cons of Remaining Attention Seeking	**Cons of Decreasing Attention Seeking**
Continued low self respect (9)	"I would miss guys attention" (8)
Continued fake relationships (10)	I would lose a bit of myself (7)
Run off "good" guys (10)	Might hurt career (5)

Results:

__11__ Reasons to remain attention seeking

__15__ Reasons to decrease attention seeking

__29__ Reasons to not remain attention seeking

__20__ Reasons to not reduce attention seeking

My Conclusions: I want guys' attention, but I'd like to have the attention of a different type of guy

I want to climb the ladder, but I'm not sure of the best way to do it

My Commitments: I will tell Rob I cannot see him anymore

I will go to the Seminar on "Real Relationships" being offered in the community

My Pros and Cons of Attention-Seeking Behavior

Pros of Remaining Attention-Seeking	Pros of Decreasing Attention Seeking

Cons of Remaining Attention Seeking	Cons of Decreasing Attention Seeking

Results:

_____ Reasons to remain attention seeking

_____ Reasons to not stay attention seeking

_____ Reasons to reduce attention seeking

_____ Reasons to not reduce attention seeking

My Conclusions _____

_____

_____

My Commitment(s) _____
_____
_____
_____
_____

Tool #4: Identify Behavioral Targets

HPD manifests differently in different people. While all present in dramatic and attention seeking ways, there are two primary areas of potential behavioral targets. The first has to do with physical appearance. In this area, flirting, sexual advances, flattery, excessive touching, and sexual promiscuity are common manifestations. A second area has to do with physical symptoms or body related complaints. Somatic conditions, feigning, or other "sicknesses" can be a part of the clinical presentation. Over-focus on a particular body part is not rare either (i.e., breasts, thighs, wrinkles, etc.—some area that has a real or perceived affect on the person's attractiveness).

Use this tool to identify some of your histrionic behaviors that you or others have noticed. Feel free to use any of the above behaviors that fit you, or list some of your own.

- **Behaviors related to my attention-seeking or impulsivity traits that I or someone else identified which I am willing to target to improve my situation**

    1. _____
    2. _____
    3. _____
    4. _____
    5. _____

Tool #5: Intimacy Circles

Intimacy is a scary word for a lot of people. If the sound of it makes you cringe, this exercise is definitely for you—and even if it doesn't, this exercise likely will still benefit you. It will benefit almost everyone in some way. Why? Because almost everyone could benefit from improving at least one interpersonal relationship in their life. Some people's lives could be enriched with more friends. Others need to learn to set boundaries with someone in their life. A lot of people have "trust issues." Yet others would be happier in life if they learned to pick healthier people to date or form friendships with; toxic people have a way of draining people of their energy and joy. A certain percentage of the population would be much less prone to mood swings if they could be okay alone. Some would find more fulfillment in life if they could share more with people in their lives; others would not be hurt as often if they learned to share less with those in their life. A lot of people walk around with their "walls" up. Some have difficulty expressing feelings. Some have been accused of being too "needy." Others have difficulty asking for help.

You may have heard intimacy defined as "Into-Me-See"——the degree to which we let people see into us, and vice versa. A lot of my clients have found this "play on words" to be a helpful way to remember its definition and connotations.

Use the following tool to evaluate the relationships in your life. Use the percentage signs to help you decide which people to put in which circles. No other person goes in the ME circle (though some people choose to put God here). This is for you alone. People who belong in circle #1 are those with whom you would feel comfortable sharing ANY problem in life, no matter how personal (a sexual problem, something related to an abusive situation, a salary issue, etc.). People in circle #2 are those in your life with whom there may be a personal issue or two (like the ones mentioned above) that you would not share, but you would be comfortable sharing ALMOST anything (roughly 75%) about your life. People in circle #3 may get about half of your personal stuff, but the other half you probably would not trust them with. People in circle #4 would be your very casual relationships. Maybe they know whether you are married or where you work or something of that nature, but you don't share very much with them (roughly 25%). And people in circle #5 get nothing. For some people, these are individuals whom they have just met, so they could be candidates to move closer in as they get to know them. Or, these are people who at one point in life were closer in, but they have done something to violate trust, so they have had to be moved out one or more rings.

This exercise will likely be difficult for you if you have histrionic traits, but those who follow through with it will reap the most meaningful rewards. Consider how close you really are to your significant others, family, and friends, and whether you consider those relationships to make you healthier and happier. Take a hard look at what your interactions look like.

Keep these ideas in mind as you consider who truly belongs where as you complete your circles. Your first task is to think about all the people in your life and where they go in your circles. Then consider the questions that follow. Whether you are able to use this to improve your own relationships or to help someone else in your life, I hope you find it to be a useful tool.

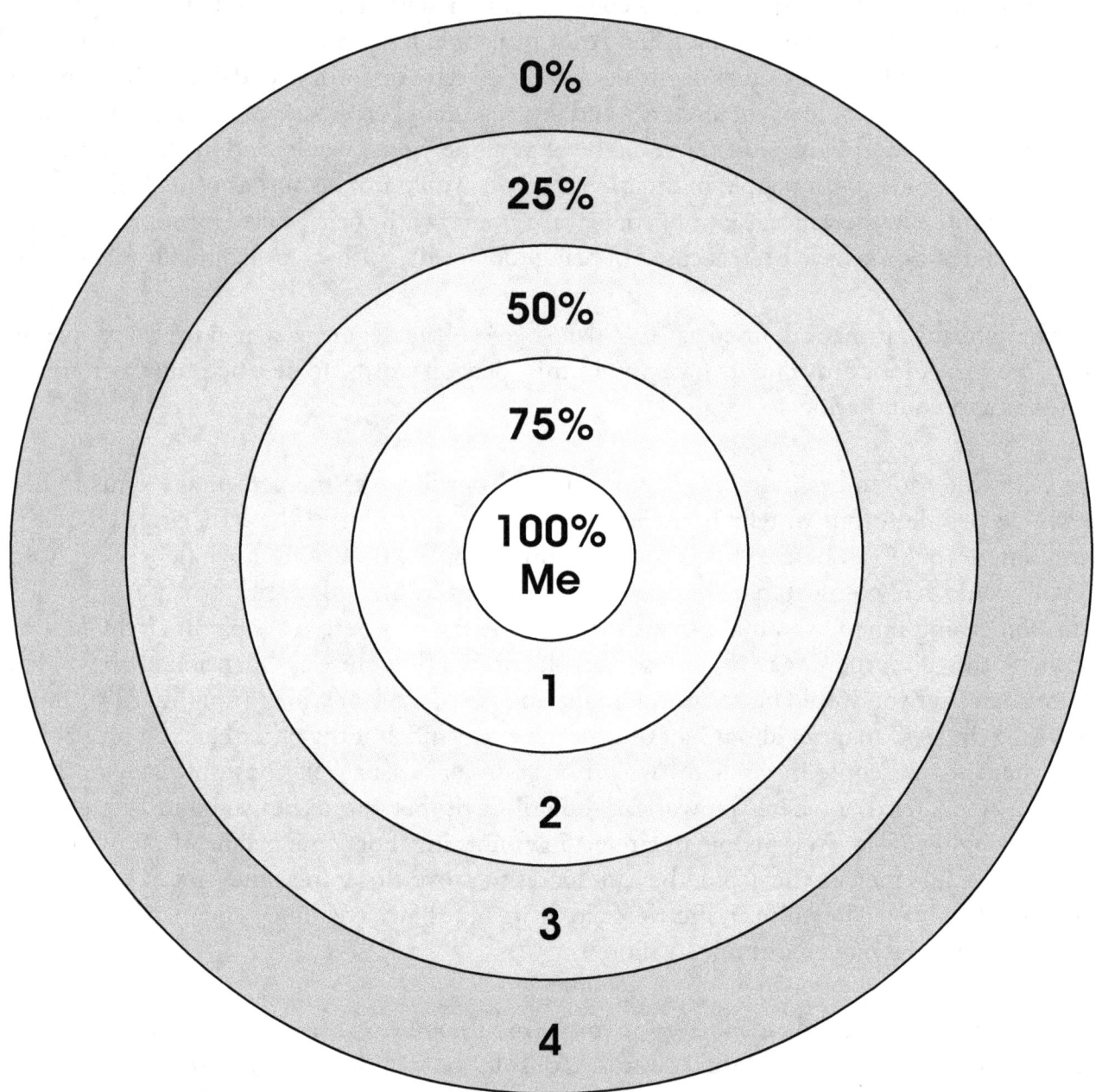

Intimacy Circles Follow-Up Starter Questions

- General observations about my circles _____
_____
_____

- What I like most about my circles _____
  _____
  _____
  _____

- What I like least about my circles _____
  _____
  _____
  _____

- The most problematic people in my life _____
  _____
  _____
  _____

- They are problematic in the following ways _____
  _____
  _____
  _____

- People in my life whose opinions I actually care about and on a scale of 0-10 how much I care what they think _____
  _____
  _____
  _____

- People in my life whose opinions I don't care about _____
  _____
  _____

Chapter 5: The Histrionic Personality Disorder

- People in my life whom I have hurt/violated/taken advantage of _____
  _____
  _____
  _____

- People in my life who have moved themselves out in my circles due to my behavior
  _____
  _____
  _____
  _____

- I could improve my circles if I were willing to keep the following rules (which I have not previously been willing to keep) _____
  _____
  _____
  _____

- One step I will take TODAY to improve my relationship circles _____
  _____
  _____
  _____

Tool #6: Identify and Restructure Automatic Thoughts

A staple component of treatment for any psychological condition is recognizing the thought processes that are driving the problem behaviors and maintaining the symptoms. In colloquial language, you may hear this referred to as "self-talk." To speak in the terms of the Mark Twain quote in the introduction ("If all you have is a hammer, everything looks like a nail"): This is the "hammer." While treatment of personality disorders requires more tools than just a hammer, the hammer is still a useful tool to have in your toolbox.

Some people develop an awareness of their thoughts and get better at noticing them, but do nothing to change them; for example, if we recognize that we are overweight, but do nothing to change our diets or exercise levels, we will stay overweight. In the same way, if we recognize thoughts that are driving problem behavior but do nothing to change them, our symptoms are likely to remain.

So, one cognitive tool you can use is what is called *challenging distorted thoughts* when you recognize them. Refer to the beginning of this chapter for some distorted thoughts common in avoidant personality disorder. *"Challenging,"* in this case, basically means arguing with the specific content of the thoughts. There are a number of techniques that can be used for doing this, including looking at evidence, seeking input from others, researching the facts, considering past or possible future results, accepting, or good old-fashioned logic, just to name a few.

The following tool asks you to identify specific attention-seeking thoughts that enter your mind, challenge them in some way, and if you want to, rate your challenge on a scale of 0-10 to indicate how meaningful the struggle is. Take a look at the example, and then do one on your own. This may be a tool that you benefit from using on an ongoing basis.

Example: Thought Log

Dramatic Thought	Rational Responses
If I can get five men to ask for my number, it will be a good night	Based upon my past relationships, I should be concerned with quality over quantity So what if five people ask? How will my life be better tomorrow? Some of these guys I'd rather not even talk to Does it matter why they ask for my number? Since most guys want to hook up with me, I might as well get the attention of someone who actually likes me

Analysis: This female client mentioned in a session that she was offended that her friend had criticized her for saying this as they walked into a club earlier in the week. This opened a discussion to look at alternative ways of thinking about herself and her life as she went out at night. She was able to identify first and foremost the tumultuous nature of her prior relationships, and this led to a fairly in-depth (for her) chat about what makes someone valuable. This set us up for evidence log work moving forward.

My Histrionic Thought Log

Dramatic Thought	Rational Responses

Tool #7: Historical Experiences Worksheet

As with most, if not all, personality disorders, there are multiple pathways to HPD. Although it is known that HPD has at least a mild genetic component, many people with these traits do have some commonalities in their backgrounds of experience. However, as with some other PDs, there is little professional research in this area. Peruse the following historical experiences that have been reported with this disorder and put an "X" beside factors that were a part of your experiences from a young age.

- ❏ History of being ignored
- ❏ History of not getting needs met
- ❏ Parents were absent
- ❏ Parents were preoccupied or self-centered
- ❏ In-depth conversation was avoided
- ❏ Surface-level conversation was rewarded
- ❏ Physical beauty was emphasized
- ❏ "Ugly" people were devalued
- ❏ Had large number of siblings and getting a parent's attention required extreme measures

- Describe how the experiences checked above applies specifically to you and the impact you believe they continue to make in your life today

_____
_____
_____
_____
_____
_____
_____
_____
_____
_____
_____
_____

Tool #8: Belief Identification

As has been discussed, all behaviors are a product of beliefs. Beliefs drive behavior. Due to the compelling nature of beliefs in individuals with PDs, these deeper-level beliefs often have to be modified to help create lasting change. As noted at the beginning of this chapter, common beliefs in people with HPD include defectiveness, approval seeking, emotional inhibition (overcompensating style), and insufficient self-control. Review their definitions if you don't have them fresh in your mind. Get with your therapist.

Include friends and family who are willing to give you feedback. Identify one or two beliefs that you believe drive your target behaviors to work on in treatment. Write them inside Judy Beck's "Pac-Man" visual aid (which was explained in the introduction).

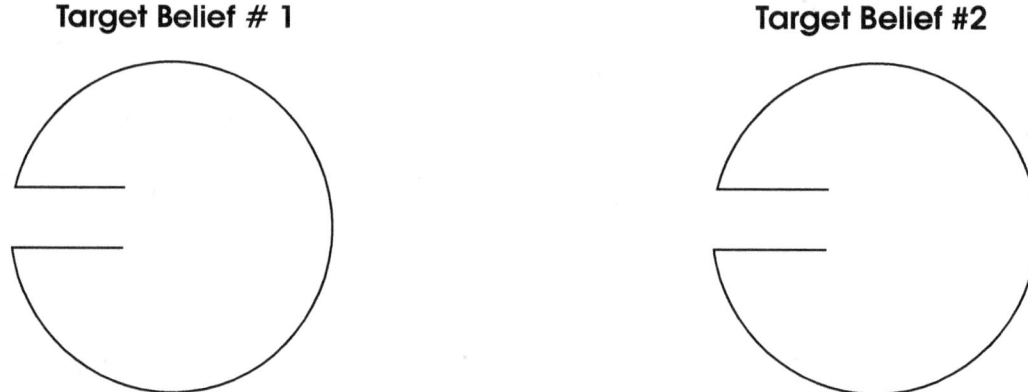

Beliefs always come in pairs. For every maladaptive (or unhealthy) belief we possess, we also possess an alternate, adaptive (or healthy) belief. For instance, if one has the belief, "I must garner men's attention to be somebody/have worth" the opposite belief we would want to cultivate would be something like, "I have value regardless of the attention I get."

I have given you the "pushing buttons" language, the "Pac-Man" visual, and the "filters" imagery. Here is another representation which I hope helps illustrate the point: We could think of beliefs as lenses. For people who wear glasses, this visual probably comes fairly intuitively. Healthier individuals are able to engage in more balanced information processing. Figuratively speaking they are able to see out of both the left and the right "lenses" equally. This is the goal of belief modification work: balanced information processing. In other words, to be able to see both sides objectively and to be able to recognize when they fail or make mistakes, so they can learn from them; and also to be able to acknowledge when they succeed and be able to take a compliment. Although nobody is perfect and everyone has their biases, healthier people's lenses are closer to the 50/50 range (50% failure/50% success). Before treatment, people with PDs, due to their more compelling beliefs, often start with numbers such as 99%/1%. ***Intentional and sustained effort*** is required to create a healthier belief balance.

So, now that you have identified your unhealthy beliefs driving your target behaviors, identify, in your own words, what you would call the opposite, healthy belief. Write it in the opposite belief structure that the "triangle" could fit into.

After you have identified your one or two healthy and unhealthy beliefs, ask your self: What percentage of the time do I believe the unhealthy belief? What percentage of the time do I believe the healthy belief? Write your numbers in the line next to each belief. (they should total 100%). Then you are ready to move on to Tool #9!

See the example first, and then do one on your own!

Example: Belief Identification

Target Belief #1	Healthy Belief #1
"Worthless Unless Attractive"	"Have Value Regardless of Appearance"
90% Strength	10% Strength

Target Belief #2	Healthy Belief #2
Strength	Strength

My Beliefs

Target Belief #1	Healthy Belief #1
Strength	Strength
Target Belief #2	**Healthy Belief #2**
Strength	Strength

Tool #9: Evidence Logs

Here is where the hard work begins! This is a tool you will use throughout your treatment, regardless of what other tools you may be using and at what stage of treatment you may be at. This is the tough, tough work of gradually working to develop your healthy belief. How do we change beliefs, anyway? It's a difficult process, no doubt. What we need to do is to *reexamine historical evidence*, *get better at noticing current evidence* **and** *intentionality initiate ongoing experiences around which to create new evidence*.

Think of any belief that you have changed over time in any area of your life. Maybe you used to not believe in God and now you do. Perhaps you used to not believe in global warming and now you do. Maybe you used to believe in life on other planets and now you don't. For example, I have a client who is a marine biology major in college – his chief interest is in Megalodon sharks, which he was initially convinced were not extinct. After a lot of scientific research, he now no longer believes that. Did you used to hold more conservative political beliefs, and your beliefs are now more progressive? You get the gist. You can use a belief that you have changed in any area of life to illustrate this process. How do

beliefs change? By examining the evidence created by experience and the meaning that we assign to it.

Take a belief many people once held. (WARNING! UPCOMING CONTENT NOT APPROPRIATE FOR KIDS!) Santa Claus is not real. If you believed in his existence when you were six years old, what was the "evidence" that supported your belief? He brought presents. They said "from Santa" on the wrapping. He drank the milk that was set out for him. He knew what presents were desired from the letters that was sent to him at the North Pole. The local weather even tracks him on the Doppler radar!

Over time, most people reexamine the pieces of evidence and assign new meaning to them. By doing so, they change their belief.

But they have to *experience* new evidence.

Some children recognize Papa beneath the Santa suit and false white beard. Some children stay up all night and sneak downstairs to catch a parent putting presents under the tree. Some children are observant enough to notice that "Santa" has Mommy's identical hand writing or wrapping paper. The child who does *not* go out of their way to look for these things holds onto the old, false belief much longer because they are not looking for evidence to the contrary. In fact, when I myself was becoming suspicious but desperately wanted to believe that he was real as a child, I began actively searching out confirmation of his existence.

In the same way, for any of us to change our beliefs, we must be *willing* to examine evidence fairly. We are naturally (consciously or unconsciously) looking for evidence to support our existing belief. But we must be equally willing to consider evidence to the contrary as well. This is what the evidence logs do: they provide a tool to facilitate *purposefully looking for evidence* to support the new belief you are attempting to construct. If your current unhealthy belief is that you are a failure, then you are purposefully looking for evidence that you can succeed. For some cognitive behavioral therapy (CBT) exercises, we will ask people to log evidence on *both* sides. But because people with PDs have such deeply engrained beliefs, their natural tendency will be to see only evidence that supports the current belief. So, for the purpose of this exercise, it is important to use the right column only to log evidence that supports the belief. The left column will remain blank.

As you record the evidence, think about how it felt to have that experience. As you do, ask yourself: *In this moment* how much do I believe _____ and how much do I believe _____?
　　　　　　　　　　　　　　　　　(unhealthy belief)　　　　　　　　　　　　　　(healthy belief)

Remember, you will inherently *not notice* evidence that will be helpful because your filter is directing you away from it, so be vigilant. Also, when you log evidence for a healthy belief, you will get that little voice in your head that says, "but… it doesn't count because of this or that." Go ahead and record the evidence anyway even if you have trouble believing it at the time.

Log the believability rating as you record each piece of evidence. Note that these numbers will go up

and down, because beliefs fluctuate. But over time, watch your unhealthy numbers generally trend down and your healthy numbers trend up. The more they change, the more balanced your lenses will be come and you will get your "buttons pushed" less frequently!

Look at the example below. Then begin completing your own evidence log, working on one belief at a time. When you have more than one icebergs to conquer, the more effort you put into chiseling one at a time, the more progress you will make.

Example: Evidence Log

Unhealthy Belief: 90%   Healthy Belief: 10%

Date	"Worthless Unless Attractive"	% Belief	"Have Value Regardless of Appearance"	% Belief
5/9		90%	Didn't intrude when Meg was talking to hot guy at bar	25%
5/11		85%	Talked to guy without flirting or touching at the social	20%
5/13		50%	Volunteered at kids' field trip for school; – had not contact with men and – just helped kids	45%
5/15		60%	Helped with kids' reading program	30%
5/17		60%	Girl Scout trip	40%

Conclusions: Even though it is hard to resist an urge to approach a man, I am starting to notice having some genuine satisfaction, at least for a few moments, helping kids

My Evidence Log

Unhealthy Belief: **Healthy Belief:**

Date		% Belief		% Belief

Conclusions _____

_____

Tool #10: Get Noticed!

People with histrionic traits have a need to be the center of attention and are triggered most often by romantic related interests not noticing them. Use the following tool to explore your need to be noticed.

- I typically notice others most when _____

- Qualities that make me notice other people most often are
    1. _____
    2. _____
    3. _____

- It is most important for me to be noticed by _____

- When I get noticed by the person I want, I feel _____

- When I am not noticed by someone who I am hoping to get their attention, I feel _____

- I think others notice me most when _____

- I think others notice me because _____

- I think this strategy of being the center of attention has affected me in the following ways _____
_____
_____

Tool #11: Star in Your Own Drama (Sculpting Tool)

My favorite genre of movie is dramas. Way back in the day when they had video rental stores (yes, I am old) I would walk in and head straight to the drama section. I think most people love a good drama.

However, for people with histrionic traits, drama can be a way of life. Although it can create painful outcomes in life of which they often lack awareness, there is also something exciting about it.

This tool will allow you to harness your dramatic flare to bolster your recovery. For maximum benefit, however, this tool requires others in your life to play along as well. If they don't, you can still benefit—it just won't be as fun.

The first step is to get out your circles from Tool #5. Identify one to four people in your circle that you would call your closest friends or family members. Ask them (or have your therapist ask them) if they will come in for a joint session to support your treatment efforts. If they don't agree, ask them if they are at least willing to fill out a brief worksheet about them and have a conversation with you about it.

Set up a time to discuss it with them. If they give you honest feedback, you might not like a few of the answers you get. This will be uncomfortable, but it's all part of the growth process.

If they do agree to come in, tell them your therapist will be sending them a questionnaire to fill out beforehand. It is important that you don't see their answers before the joint session. Here is the form:

Perception of Closeness Tool

- What did you think of me when you first met me?
- What is your spouse's opinion of me?
- What are your friend's opinion of me?
- What do others in the family think of me?
- What do you admire in me?
- What do you not like about me?
- What do you notice about me when we go out together?
- Are there reasons you think other people don't respect me? If so, What?
- On a scale of 0-10, how close do you view our relationship?
- Why from your perspective aren't we closer?
- Is there anything I can do to help improve our relationship?

During your joint session, your therapist can use the form as a guide to facilitate an exercise called ***sculpting***. Sculpting was made popular by Virginia Satir and other family therapists back in the 1980s. It is especially powerful for assessing family dynamics, but can be equally useful for people with PDs, for different reasons.

Therapist's Sculpting Guide

First, explain sculpting. If you aren't familiar with it, a brief explanation might sound something like this:

I want you to pretend like you are a sculptor, and the characters in the scene of this drama are made of clay. You can place them in any position you want in order to represent your relationship to them. Hands can be up or down; they can be touching each other or on the other side of the room. They can be facing each other or looking away. They can be standing on chairs. They can have different facial expressions. You are the director of this scene.

Something like that usually will suffice. Answer any questions, and then begin.

1. Start by having the patient sculpt how they view the relationship to their support person. Guide them as needed. Questions might include:

- Where would they go in the room?

- Which direction would you like them to face?

- What is their posture like?

2. Once you have seen the patient's perception, use the guideline sheet to facilitate the same process from the support person's perspective. Guide them in a similar way.

3. Point out differences in perception of closeness. Ask the patient questions like:

- Did you have any idea they would set the scene like this?

- How does it feel that they have you in that position relative to them?

- What is different about your scene versus their scene?

- Now that you have seen what your perception is versus what their perception is, how would you like the scene to change? (Allow patient to sculpt desired change in scene)

4. Tell the patient to ask the other if that scene is possible. Facilitate the discussion and develop action steps. Follow up as indicated.

Tool #12: Identifying Needs

At the beginning of this chapter it is mentioned that individuals with histrionic traits typically have emotional deprivation schemas. You may remember that such schemas are related to unmet needs.

Use the following tool to identify needs that you have in different areas. You may discount some of these initially, but please double down on your efforts to hear your therapist's feedback on this one. To the left of each, rate on a scale of 0-10 how important that particular need is to you.

Needs Checklist Tool

- ❏ Feeling Accepted
- ❏ Not Being Judged
- ❏ Education
- ❏ Approval
- ❏ Being Appreciated
- ❏ Sense of Belonging
- ❏ Feeling Accomplished
- ❏ Feeling Valued
- ❏ Connectedness
- ❏ To be challenged
- ❏ Food/Water/Shelter
- ❏ Autonomy

- ❏ Knowledge
- ❏ Conscientiousness
- ❏ To be in control
- ❏ Empowered
- ❏ To get attention
- ❏ To be useful to society
- ❏ Feeling Admired
- ❏ Respect
- ❏ Education
- ❏ Openness
- ❏ To do things right
- ❏ Personal Growth

Tool #13: Getting Needs Met Appropriately Tool

If you did the tool above, great job! It can be a challenge for many people with histrionic traits to even be able to identify their needs. Also, many attempt to get needs met in inappropriate ways which lead to the problems that land them in treatment. This tool will pick up where the previous one left off by helping you to clarify what the "need" means to you, who in your life is appropriate to meet that need, and how to go about getting it met.

Example:

Need	What it Means to Me	Who in My Circles is Appropriate To Meet it	What I Need to do to Get it Met
Connectedness	1. Having someone to call for emotional support 2. Physical affection 3. Sexual contact	1. Mom, aunt, sister 2. Mom, friend Amy 3. Nobody right now—I need to wait to get this need met	1. Ask 2. Explain to them what I am working on 3. Find a man that will treat me well

My Need	What it Means to Me	Who in My Circles is Appropriate To Meet it	What I Need to do to Get it Met
1.	1. 2. 3.	1. 2. 3.	1. 2. 3.
1.	1. 2. 3.	1. 2. 3.	1. 2. 3.

My Conclusions _____

Tool #14: Expanding My Self-Worth

As previously mentioned, people with histrionic traits value physical appearance above all else. There is nothing wrong with valuing physical attraction and—even more so—the healthy lifestyle that is part of maintaining it. Problems can present themselves, however, when this is the most important thing in our mind. Relationships crumble, conversation can be superficial, and life often lacks depth and meaning.

Another by-product is that depression rates seem to skyrocket in people with HPD around the age of fifty. Father Time catches up with us all, and none of us look like we are twenty when we are fifty. Nobody likes this fact, but most people come to accept it. This is, of course, easier accomplished when one values other things in life more than (or at least as much as) physical attractiveness. If looking beautiful is all that one values and age begins to rob them of that, many of these individuals are crushed. Some go to drastic measures to maintain their appearance as long as possible, going so far as to take harmful medications, have multiple plastic surgeries (which can be harmful), and even develop eating disorders and related medical complications.

If this describes you, use this tool to try to identify some things you can start to value in addition to physical attractiveness. Think in terms of spirituality and faith, hobbies, values, causes that are important to you, etc. Tool #13 dealing with identity in the chapter on dependent personality disorder may be useful to help you explore this as well.

- Five things I could try to get involved with that I value in addition to my looks

    1. _____
    2. _____
    3. _____
    4. _____
    5. _____

Tool #15: Making Meaningful Connections

There almost shouldn't be a tool for this one. But this is a toolbox. And histrionic (as well as narcissistic) individuals have difficulty with this. While there is little to describe, the application can be difficult and it requires consistent work over time, not to mention a willingness to share the attention in the conversation as well as to go deep, which does not come natural for you if you have this particular set of personality traits. It simply involves building an authentic relationship with someone—hopefully, eventually, more than one someone. But we all have to start somewhere. Use the following tool to facilitate this process for yourself.

- The person in my life I am willing to try to "go deep" with _____

- I commit to meet with them _____
  (how often?)

- I have known that person for the following length of time _____

- I know the following things about them _____
_____
_____

- I commit to being cognizant of time and allowing them to share with me as well. I will monitor my responses and attempt to be supportive. When they give me a compliment or attempt to meet one of my needs, I will make every attempt to receive it, even if it is uncomfortable.

- Some things I look forward to learning about them _____
_____
_____

- Some questions I will ask them _____
_____
_____

- Some compliments they may give me or needs I have which they may attempt to meet, which will be uncomfortable for me _____
_____
_____

- Some values we have in common which we can discuss _____
_____
_____

Chapter 5: The Histrionic Personality Disorder

- Some hobbies we have in common which we can discuss _____
_____
_____

- When I am tempted to cancel a meeting or walk away from the relationship, here are some things I can remind myself of _____
_____

- Questions or comments I have for my therapist as I embark on this journey _____
_____
_____
_____
_____
_____

CHAPTER 6:
THE ANTISOCIAL PERSONALITY DISORDER

The Antisocial Personality Disorder

Hidden agenda: To get what they want (instant gratification)

Prevalence rates: 3-4% of the general population

Gender distribution: Significantly more common in men than women

Cognitive profile:

- View of self: "I am strong," "I must stay autonomous"

- View of others: "Others are vulnerable," Others are to be exploited"

- View of world: "The world is to be violated/exploited"

Common schemas: Social isolation, punitiveness, subjugation, entitlement, insufficient self-control

Common cognitive distortions: Rationalization, "should" statements (directed towards others)

Overdeveloped traits: Combativeness, exploitiveness

Underdeveloped traits: Reciprocity, social sensitivity

Whom they date/marry: Dependents

Where they work: Drug dealers, criminal enterprises, manual labor, corporate America, sales

Other Random Nuggets: It has been estimated that a third of individuals with antisocial personality disorder (ASPD) qualify as psychopaths

Continuum

Mild — **Moderate** — **Severe**

Mild	Moderate	Severe
Disregard for societal norms	Mild run-ins with the law	Hurts or kills people with no remorse
Breaks rules	Verbal and/or Physical Violence	Callous and unemotional
Indifferent to criticism	Short stints in jail	Higher criminal lever activity
		Higher security level incarcerations when caught

Tool #1: Trait Checklist

Individuals that suffer from the characteristics of antisocial personality disorder (ASPD) have a number of commonalities. Whether you are a loved one has this full blown condition, or some of the traits of it, survey the following checklist. The more of these you check yes to, the more likely it is this pattern of behavior is causing some problems occupationally, relationally, or socially.

- ❏ Shows a pattern of disrespect toward society's norms, expectations, or rules

- ❏ Oftentimes has a history of run-ins with the law or engagement in illegal behavior without being caught

- ❏ Can be extremely charming on the surface level

- ❏ Takes advantage of people in callous ways to get what they want

- ❏ Often plans illicit acts in premeditated and calculating ways

- ❏ Deceitful, manipulative, and dishonest to get what they want

- ❏ Feels little to no remorse regardless how heinous an act of violence may have been

- ❏ Can be impulsive with alcohol, drugs, and violence

- ❏ Oftentimes puts self in harm's way

- ❏ Displays a chilling calm in situations where most people would be nervous

Tool #2: Expressions of Concern

All people have what are often called "blind spots": qualities we don't see in ourselves as well as others see in us. Because of the ego-syntonic nature of PDs, this phenomenon is particularly challenging for these people. What this means practically is that things that pose problems for friends and family members are often not are considered problematic by the individual with the condition. Concerns expressed by friends and family may have validity to them, but due to poor insight, the PD individual generally has difficulty seeing how certain behaviors impact themselves or others negatively. However, not all concerns friends and family express have validity. So, one of the tough but vital steps for recovery is sorting through these "complaints" to determine which ones have validity and which do not. One obvious problem for people with antisocial tendencies is that they don't care what others think, so feedback is rarely taken seriously. However, sometimes people with ASPD will use their charm to convince a loved one that they are taking it seriously when in reality they have no intent to change their behavior.

Use the following tool to identify *who* has expressed concern, *what* the exact concerns are, and *why* they see them as potentially hurtful. Look at the example, then complete your own and answer the questions that follow.

Example:

Person Expressing Concern	Action Causing Concern	Reason for Concern
1. Girlfriend	1. Using again immediately after release	1. Possible reincarceration
2. Parole officer	2. Absent for meetings	2. Possible reincarceration
3. Daughter	3. Not coming home in the evenings	3. Don't know if I am "okay"
4. Sponsor	4. Using again; hanging out with the wrong people	4. Possible reincarceration; general fear for safety and well-being

Questions:

- Who are three people I trust to "shoot straight" with me, by whom I can run these concerns to get their opinion?

    1. My buddy Charlie

    2. ?

    3. ?

- With which concerns can I at least see where the person is coming from?

    It's more likely that I'll go back than die—I can take care of myself. But my daughter is the only person I care about

- Which concerns can I see the most validity in?

    ?

- I am willing to take the following steps to change one of the concerns:

    1. Take extra precautions not to get caught—change where I party

    2. Not miss any more meetings with parole officer

    3. ?

My Expressions of Concern

Person Expressing Concern	Action Causing Concern	Reason for Concern
1.	1.	1.
2.	2.	2.
3.	3.	3.
4.	4.	4.
5.	5.	5.

Questions:

- Who are three people I trust to "shoot straight" with me, by whom I can run these concerns by to get their opinion?

    1. _____

    2. _____

    3. _____

- With which concerns can I at least see where the person is coming from? _____
  _____
  _____

- Which concerns can I see the most validity in? _____
  _____
  _____

- I am willing to take the following steps to change one of the concerns
    1. _____
    2. _____
    3. _____

Tool #3: Pros and Cons

This tool helps you evaluate the potential pros and cons of your rule-breaking behaviors. It is called a *four-box pros and cons*. Sometimes it can be beneficial to look at not only the advantages and disadvantages of maintaining certain behaviors but also the advantages and disadvantages of changing them. After listing the pros and cons of each, it can be even more helpful to rate, on a scale of 0-10, how important each item is. Consider the example that is provided. Then complete one on your own!

Example: Pros and Cons of Rule-Breaking Behavior

Pros of Rule-Breaking Behavior	Pros of Keeping Rules
Get what I want (7)	Keep strong relationship with daughter (10)
Stay in charge (8)	Keep a job/make money (7)
Don't have to answer to anybody (5)	Cops stop watching me (5)
Cons of of Rule-Breaking Behavior	**Cons of Keeping Rules**
Did time (10)	Not as fun (7)
Lost relationship with daughter (10)	Life is boring (7)

Results:

__20__ Reasons to continue rule breaking behaviors

__20__ Reasons to stop rule breaking behavior

__22__ Reasons to keep the rules/laws

__14__ Reasons not to break rules

My Conclusions They were closer than I thought

My Commitment Keep all my appointments with my PO and walk straight

My Pros and Cons of Antisocial Behavior

Pros of Rule-Breaking Behavior	Pros of Keeping Rules
Cons of Rule-Breaking Behavior	Cons of Keeping Rules

Results:

_____ Reasons to keep rule-breaking

_____ Reasons to not keep rule-breaking

_____ Reasons to reduce keep rule-breaking

_____ Reasons to not reduce keep rule-breaking

My Conclusions _____
_____
_____
_____

My Commitment(s) _____
_____
_____
_____
_____

Tool #4: Identify Behavioral Targets

Antisocial personality traits manifest differently in different people. Milder behaviors include lying, petty theft, mild manipulative or controlling behavior, and thrill-seeking behaviors. They often commit minor law-breaking violations (i.e., speeding, marijuana use, stealing from restaurants or small items from stores). Common behaviors include verbal or physical violence, regular substance use, gang related involvement, or other criminal activity. More extreme manifestations, which may qualify as *psychopathic* behaviors, include large-scale robbery, cruelty to animals, regular physical violence, rape, murder, and other extreme behaviors that hurt society as well as individuals in a very callous way, with no remorse whatsoever.

Use this tool to identify some of your antisocial behaviors that you or others have noticed. Feel free to use any of the above behaviors that fit, or list some of your own.

- Behaviors related to my antisocial traits that I or someone else identified which I am willing to target to improve my situation

1. _____
2. _____
3. _____
4. _____
5. _____

Tool #5: Intimacy Circles

Intimacy is a scary word for a lot of people. If the sound of it makes you cringe, this exercise is definitely for you—and even if it doesn't, this exercise likely will still benefit you. It will benefit almost everyone in some way. Why? Because almost everyone could benefit from improving at least one interpersonal relationship in their life. Some people's lives could be enriched with more friends. Others need to learn to set boundaries with someone in their life. A lot of people have "trust issues." Yet others would be happier in life if they learned to pick healthier people to date or form friendships with; toxic people have a way of draining people of their energy and joy. A certain percentage of the population would be much less prone to mood swings if they could be okay alone. Some would find more fulfillment in life if they could share more with people in their lives; others would not be hurt as often if they learned to share less with those in their life. A lot of people walk around with their "walls" up. Some have difficulty expressing feelings. Some have been accused of being too "needy." Others have difficulty asking for help.

You may have heard intimacy defined as "Into-Me-See"——the degree to which we let people see into us, and vice versa. A lot of my clients have found this "play on words" to be a helpful way to remember its definition and connotations.

Use the following tool to evaluate the relationships in your life. Use the percentage signs to help you decide which people to put in which circles. No other person goes in the ME circle (though some people choose to put God here). This is for you alone. People who belong in circle #1 are those with whom you would feel comfortable sharing ANY problem in life, no matter how personal (a sexual problem, something related to an abusive situation, a salary issue, etc.). People in circle #2 are those in your life with whom there may be a personal issue or two (like the ones mentioned above) that you would not share, but you would be comfortable sharing ALMOST anything (roughly 75%) about your life. People in circle #3 may get about half of your personal stuff, but the other half you probably would not trust them with. People in circle #4 would be your very casual relationships. Maybe they know whether you are married or where you work or something of that nature, but you don't share very much with them (roughly 25%). And people in circle #5 get nothing. For some people, these are individuals

whom they have just met, so they could be candidates to move closer in as they get to know them. Or, these are people who at one point in life were closer in, but they have done something to violate trust, so they have had to be moved out one or more rings.

You may have heard the phrase "people need people." This is generally true. However, relationships are a bit different for most people with antisocial traits. Few attach to others to the degree that they "need" them or even care to any degree about their well-being. Some people with antisocial traits do have a central figure that they are attached to. (The serial killer who was best friends with his mom.) Also notable is the fact that people with rule-breaking tendencies have a unique ability to compartmentalize. So, for instance, if you are "one of them" (family member, fellow gang member, etc.) they will take a bullet for you; but if you are not, they may not hesitate to put a bullet in you (sometimes literally, sometimes figuratively)! The other noteworthy thing here is that quality mentioned above of superficial charm. Many individuals with ASPD have a way of coming across as extremely charming and likeable, but only superficially and usually for manipulative reasons.

Keep these ideas in mind as you consider who truly belongs where as you complete your circles. Your first task is to think about all the people in your life and where they go in your circles. Then consider the questions that follow to get you started making healthy changes to your relationships. Work with your therapist or other helping professional if you need ongoing guidance or accountability.

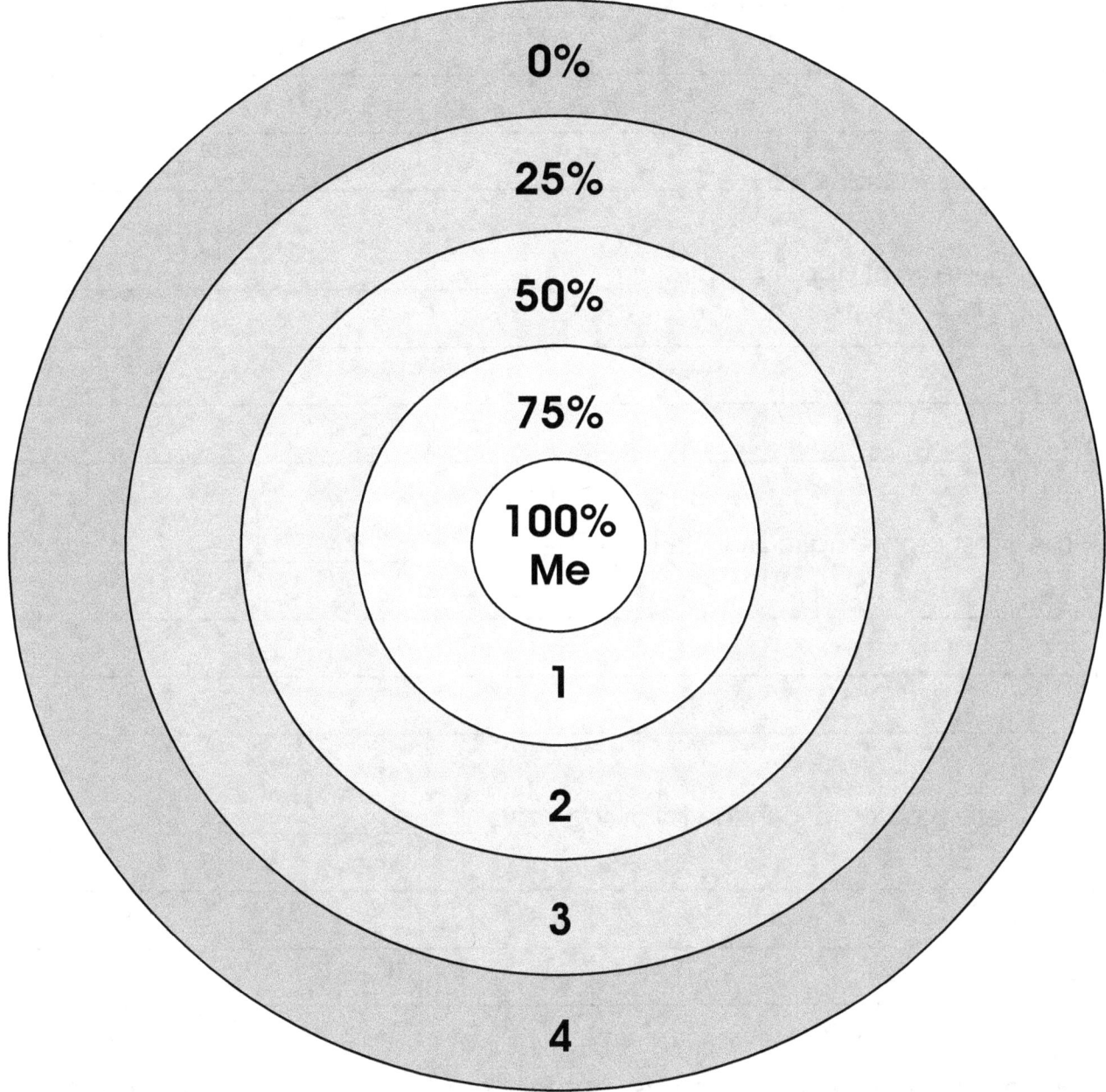

Intimacy Circles Follow-Up Starter Questions

- General observations about my circles _____
_____
_____
_____

Chapter 6: The Antisocial Personality Disorder

- What I like most about my circles _____
  _____
  _____
  _____

- What I like least about my circles _____
  _____
  _____
  _____

- The most problematic people in my life _____
  _____
  _____
  _____

- They are problematic in the following ways _____
  _____
  _____
  _____

- People in my life whose opinions I actually care about and on a scale of 0-10 how much I care what they think _____
  _____
  _____
  _____

- People in my life whose opinions I don't care about _____
  _____
  _____

- People in my life whom I have hurt/violated/taken advantage of _____
  _____
  _____
  _____

- People in my life who have moved themselves out in my circles due to my behavior
  _____
  _____
  _____
  _____

- I could improve my circles if I were willing to keep the following rules (which I have not previously been willing to keep) _____
  _____
  _____
  _____

- One step I will take TODAY to improve my relationship circles _____
  _____
  _____
  _____

Tool #6: Identify and Restructure Automatic Thoughts

A staple component of treatment for any psychological condition is recognizing the thought processes that are driving the problem behaviors and maintaining the symptoms. In colloquial language, you may hear this referred to as "self-talk." To speak in the terms of the Mark Twain quote in the introduction ("If all you have is a hammer, everything looks like a nail"): This is the "hammer." While treatment of personality disorders requires more tools than just a hammer, the hammer is still a useful tool to have in your toolbox.

Some people develop an awareness of their thoughts and get better at noticing them, but do nothing to change them. For example, if we recognize that we are overweight, but do nothing to change our diets

or exercise levels, we will stay overweight. In the same way, if we recognize thoughts that are driving problem behavior but do nothing to change them, our symptoms are likely to remain.

So, one cognitive tool you can use is what is called challenging distorted thoughts when you recognize them. Refer to the beginning of this chapter for some distorted thoughts common in antisocial personality disorder. *"Challenging,"* in this case, basically means "arguing" with the specific content of the thoughts. There are a number of techniques that can be used for doing this, including looking at evidence, seeking input from others, researching the facts, considering past or possible future results, or good old-fashioned logic, just to name a few.

The following tool asks you to identify specific antisocial thoughts that enter your mind, challenge them in some way, and if you want to, rate your challenge on a scale of 0-10, indicating how meaningful the challenge is. Take a look at the example, and then do one on your own. This may be a tool that you will benefit from using on an ongoing basis.

Example: Thought Log

Rule-Breaking Thoughts	Rational Responses
It was okay to rob the store because I wanted the electronics. My family deserves them as much as anyone else	It's not okay because it's not right (1) It's not a good idea because I might get caught (5) Last time I got caught I did some time (3) We might deserve it as much as others do, but it's still not a good idea—my family needs me out (6) There are other ways to get what I want (2)

Analysis: In this instance, this particular client clearly does not care about what the right thing to do is. He makes his own rules regarding right and wrong and when they apply. He also isn't overly concerned about the prospect of doing some more time, other than that it would impact his family (mother and little brothers). Efforts to change behaviors should focus on the impact his behaviors have on them.

My Antisocial Thought Log

Rule-Breaking Thoughts	Rational Responses

Tool #7: Historical Experiences Worksheet

Its known that people with ASPD have significant brain abnormalities in comparison to people with other PDs (or those without PDs). It is not completely clear at this point what role genetics play as opposed to other factors that could influence the brain along the way. In addition to that, it is known that people with these traits do have some commonalities in their backgrounds of experience, which you may hear referred to *environmental risk factors*. Peruse the following historical experiences worksheet and put an "X" beside factors that were a part of your experiences since a young age.

- ❑ Were threatened or humiliated
- ❑ Parents who were absent
- ❑ Substance use in the family
- ❑ Gang related behavior
- ❑ Other violence in the neighborhood

- ❑ Physical or sexual abuse
- ❑ Violent behavior role modeled
- ❑ Bedwetting
- ❑ Showed cruelty to animals
- ❑ Fire setting

- Describe how the experiences checked above apply specifically to you and the impact you believe they continue to have in your life today

_____
_____
_____
_____
_____
_____
_____
_____
_____
_____

Tool #8: Belief Identification

As has been discussed, all behaviors are a product of beliefs. Beliefs drive behavior. Due to the compelling nature of beliefs in individuals with PDs, these deeper-level beliefs often have to be modified to help create lasting change. As noted at the beginning of this chapter, common beliefs in people with ASPD include social isolation, punitiveness, subjugation, entitlement, and insufficient self-control. Review their definitions if you don't have them fresh in your mind. Get with your therapist. Include friends and family who are willing to give you feedback. Identify one or two beliefs that you believe drive your target behaviors to work on in treatment. Write them inside Judy Beck's "Pac-Man" visual aid (which was explained in the introduction).

Target Belief # 1

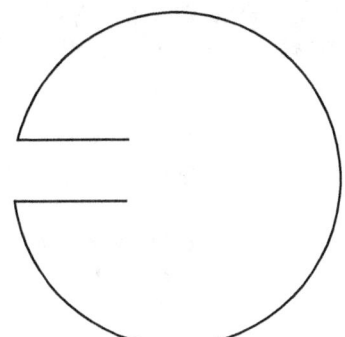

Target Belief #2

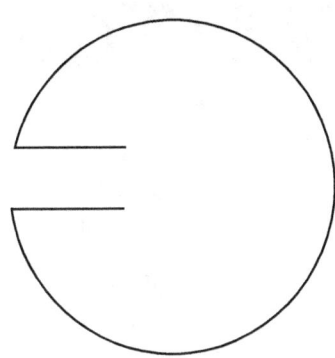

Beliefs always come in pairs. For every maladaptive (or unhealthy) belief we possess, we also possess an alternate, adaptive (or healthy) belief. For instance, even though an individual may have the belief, "I deserve to get what I want regardless of the rules," there is also the alternate belief, however faint, "It is best for me to keep the rules like others."

I have given you the "pushing buttons" language, the "Pac-Man" visual, and the "filters" imagery. Here is another representation which I hope helps illustrate the point: We could think of beliefs as lenses. For people who wear glasses, this visual probably comes fairly intuitively. Healthier individuals are able to engage in more balanced information processing. Figuratively speaking they are able to see out of both the left and the right "lenses" equally. This is the goal of belief modification work: balanced information processing. In other words, to be able to see both sides objectively and to be able to recognize when they fail or make mistakes, so they can learn from them; and also to be able to acknowledge when they succeed and be able to take a compliment. Although nobody is perfect and everyone has their biases, healthier people's lenses are closer to the 50/50 range (50% failure/50% success). Before treatment, people with PDs, due to their more compelling beliefs, often start with numbers such as 99%/1%. ***Intentional and sustained effort*** is required to create a healthier belief balance.

So, now that you have identified your unhealthy beliefs driving your target behaviors, identify in your own words what you would call the opposite, healthy belief. Write it in the opposite belief structure that the "triangle" could fit into.

After you have identified your one or two healthy and unhealthy beliefs, ask yourself: "What percentage of the time do I believe the unhealthy belief? What percentage of the time do I believe the healthy belief?" Write your numbers in the line next to each belief (they should total 100%). Then you are ready to move on to Tool #9!

See the example first, and then do one on your own!

Chapter 6: The Antisocial Personality Disorder

Example: Belief Identification

Target Belief #1	Healthy Belief #1
"I deserve to get what I want regardless of the rules"	"It is best for me to keep the rules like everybody else"
97% Strength	3% Strength
Target Belief #2	**Healthy Belief #2**
"Others are weak"	"Others deserve some respect"
95% Strength	5% Strength

My Beliefs

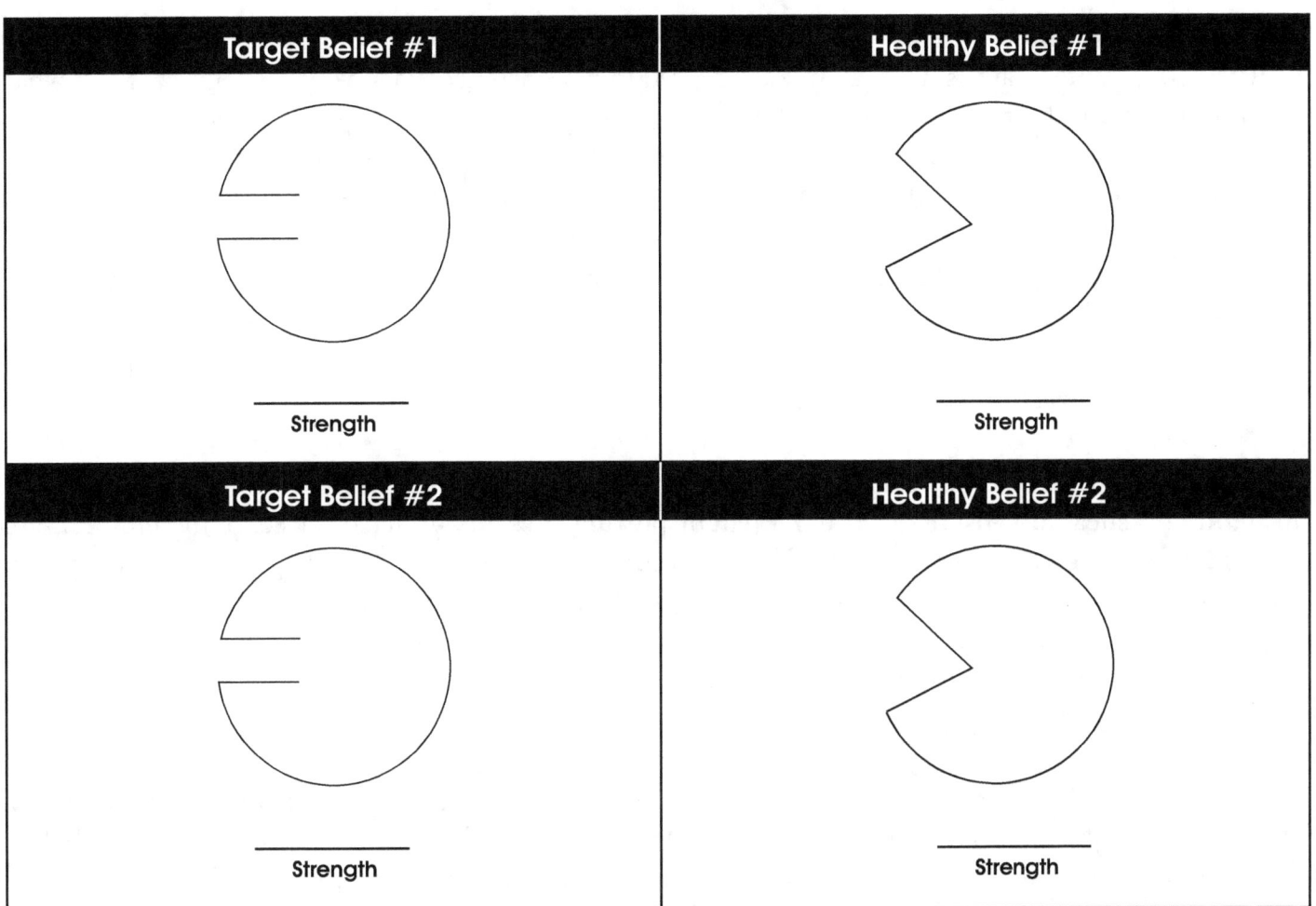

Tool #9: Evidence Logs

Here is where the hard work begins! This is a tool you will use throughout your treatment, regardless of what other tools you may be using and at what stage of treatment you may be at. This is the tough, tough work of gradually working to develop your healthy belief. How do we change beliefs, anyway? It's a difficult process, no doubt. What we need to do is to *reexamine historical evidence, get better at noticing current evidence* **and** *intentionality initiate ongoing experiences around which to create new evidence.*

Think of any belief that you have changed over time in any area of your life. Maybe you used to not believe in God and now you do. Perhaps you used to not believe in global warming and now you do. Maybe you used to believe in life on other planets and now you don't. For example, I have a client who is a marine biology major in college – his chief interest is in Megalodon sharks, which he was initially convinced were not extinct. After a lot of scientific research, he now no longer believes that. Did you used to hold more conservative political beliefs, and your beliefs are now more progressive? You get the gist. You can use a belief that you have changed in *any* area of life to illustrate this process. How do

beliefs change? By examining the evidence created by experience and the meaning that we assign to it.

Take a belief many people once held. (WARNING! UPCOMING CONTENT NOT APPROPRIATE FOR KIDS!) Santa Claus is not real. If you believed in his existence when you were six years old, what was the "evidence" that supported your belief? He brought presents. They said "from Santa" on the wrapping. He drank the milk that was set out for him. He knew what presents were desired from the letters that was sent to him at the North Pole. The local weather even tracks him on the Doppler radar!

Over time, most people reexamine the pieces of evidence and assign new meaning to them. By doing so, they change their belief.

But they have to *experience* new evidence.

Some children recognize Papa beneath the Santa suit and false white beard. Some children stay up all night and sneak downstairs to catch a parent putting presents under the tree. Some children are observant enough to notice that "Santa" has Mommy's identical hand writing or wrapping paper. The child who *does not go out of their way to look for these things* holds onto the old, false belief much longer because they are not looking for evidence to the contrary. In fact, when I myself was becoming suspicious but desperately wanted to believe that he was real as a child, I began actively searching out confirmation of his existence.

In the same way, for any of us to change our beliefs, we must be *willing* to examine evidence fairly. We are naturally (consciously or unconsciously) looking for evidence to support our existing belief. But we must be equally willing to consider evidence to the contrary as well. This is what the evidence logs do: they provide a tool to facilitate *purposefully looking for evidence* to support the new belief you are attempting to construct. If your current unhealthy belief is that you are a failure, then you are purposefully looking for evidence that you can succeed. For some cognitive behavioral therapy (CBT) exercises, we will ask people to log evidence on *both* sides. But because people with PDs have such deeply engrained beliefs, their natural tendency will be to see only evidence that supports the current belief. So, for the purpose of this exercise, it is important to use the right column only to log evidence that supports the belief. The left column will remain blank.

As you record the evidence, think about how it felt to have that experience. As you do, ask yourself: *In this moment* how much do I believe _____ and how much do I believe _____?
                                  (unhealthy belief)   (healthy belief)

Remember, you will inherently *not notice* evidence that will be helpful because your filter is directing you away from it, so be vigilant. Also, when you log evidence for a healthy belief, you will get that little voice in your head that says, "but… it doesn't count because of this or that." Go ahead and record the evidence anyway even if you have trouble believing it at the time.

Log the believability rating as you record each piece of evidence. Note that these numbers will go up

and down, because beliefs fluctuate. But over time, watch your unhealthy numbers generally trend down and your healthy numbers trend up. The more they change, the more balanced your lenses will be come and you will get your "buttons pushed" less frequently!

Look at the example below. Then begin completing your own evidence log, working on one belief at a time. When you have more than one icebergs to conquer, the more effort you put into chiseling one at a time, the more progress you will make.

Example: Evidence Log

Unhealthy Belief: 97% **Healthy Belief: 3%**

Date	"I deserve to get what I want regardless of the rules"	% Belief	"It is best for me to keep the rules like everybody else"	% Belief
10/14		97%	Stole from a convenience store, didn't get caught	3%
10/16		97%	Broke noise ordinance playing loud music till 3 a.m. and someone called the cops	3%
10/17		97%	Did illegal drugs	3%
10/18		95%	Stole from a sports store and got caught – called my parole officer	5%
10/20		95%	Resisted security guard, which caused a fight where my cousin got badly injured	5%

Conclusions Some bad shit can happen from dissing authority – you just have to call your shot, whether it's worth it

My Evidence Log

Unhealthy Belief: **Healthy Belief:**

Date		% Belief		% Belief

Conclusions _____
_____

Tool #10: Secondary Gain

Individuals with ASPD are known for their behaviors that produce secondary gain. This is generally known as an indirect benefit gained by getting sick, not solving a problem, or staying "stuck." The specific benefits themselves might include things like staying out of legal trouble, not having to complete school, receiving disability benefits, gaining access to prescription medications, or avoiding any type of unpleasant situation.

Part of treatment for any problem involves just getting honest. So, shooting completely straight, use the following tool to identify some of the specific behaviors you have engaged in (see target behaviors in Tool #4 to refresh your memory) in the past as well as the *true* motivator behind each behavior. To quote one of my clients in group therapy: "If you bullshit here, you are wasting our time."

What I Did	What I Really Hoped to Get Out of It
1.	1.
2.	2.
3.	3.

Tool #11: Recognition of Consequences and Getting What You Want

Now that it is clear that those behaviors did not cause the outcome you hoped for, let's face the facts and have an honest look at what they did get you. When I ask clients, "What did that get you?" many say, "It didn't get me anything." And my response 95% of the time is, "Yes it did. What was it?" Another way to ask this is: "What negative consequences am I currently dealing with that I would not be if hadn't done [insert target behavior]?" Use the following tool to log your responses.

What I Did	What It Really Got Me
1.	1.
2.	2.
3.	3.

Now that you have been honest, (now, how hard was that?) let's look at some alternative ways to get what you want that can spare you the consequences you don't want. Brainstorm some ways to get what you want that don't involve breaking the rules or violating people.

What I Want	Better Ways to Get it
1.	1.
2.	2.
3.	3.

The next time I want _____, instead of _____ I will
(desire) (past or typical behaviors)
_____.

Tool #12: Regaining Responsibility

Confrontations are common for people with antisocial traits. When we have an altercation of any kind, it can be difficult to assign blame.

All people do this based upon our beliefs. Due to strong beliefs and rigid, black and white thinking, people with personality disorders are unsurprisingly more prone to have difficulty doing this than others. People with certain disorder tend, however, to take on *MORE* responsibility than is rightfully theirs, while individuals with other disorders tend to take on *less* responsibility than is rightfully theirs. Also unsurprisingly, people with ASPD error on the end of the spectrum of taking LESS responsibility and blaming others for situations or aspects of situations that are in reality their fault.

Notice the term "aspects" of the situation. This is because most interactional problems in life are not all or nothing; that is they are not ALL our fault and are not ALL the other person's fault.

I remember when I was in school I would sometimes not turn in my homework. In those cases, I could usually turn it in late and still receive *Partial Credit*. This concept can be helpful for divvying up blame in confrontations or personal misunderstandings as well.

This tool gives you a chance to get "partial credit." It asks you to identify a confrontation or relational situation you have recently dealt with, assign how much of the blame/responsibility for it was yours and how much of the blame/responsibility belonged to the other person. Since your bias will likely assign more "credit" for the problem to the other person, the tool will then challenge you to consider in what way you could take a little more responsibility in the situation.

Look at the example, and then use the following tool to help assign responsibility in a shared manner.

Reclaiming Responsibility Tool

Situation: Clerk called police on me and I was escorted out of the store

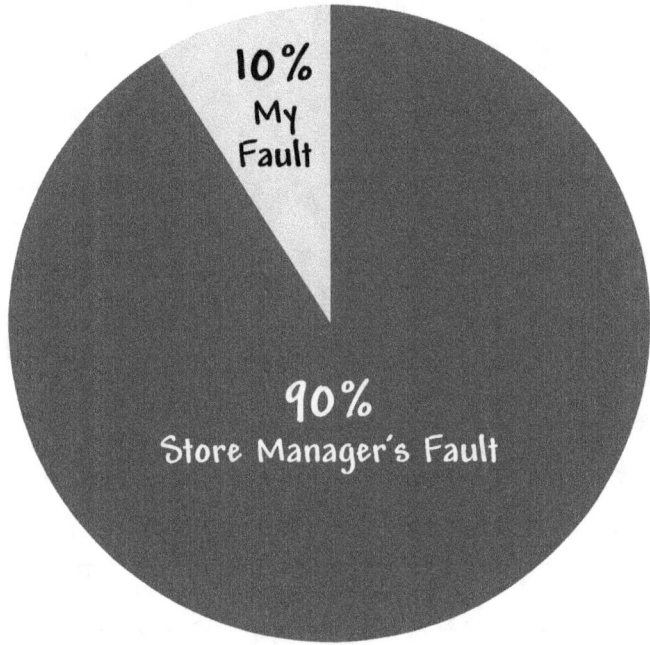

Others Responsibility: I stated that it was 90% the clerk's fault because he didn't tell me how much the item was, he didn't tell me they did not accept credit cards, he didn't help me find an alternative, he was an A-hole.

My Responsibility: I stated it was 10 % my fault because I did use a lot of profanity in front of the customers and attempt to steal it.

My Commitment:

One aspect of the situation I am willing to take responsibility for that I didn't previously is: Stealing is technically illegal

Reclaiming Responsibility Tool

Situation _____

Others Responsibility

I stated that it was ____% his/her fault because _____

_____

_____

My Responsibility

I stated it was _____ % my fault because _____

_____

_____

My Commitment

One aspect of the situation I am willing to take responsibility for that I didn't previously is _____

Tool #13: Abolishing Assumptions

Most tools up to this point have been focusing on behaviors. Most treatment available for ASPD focuses on surface-level behavioral change, since this is what keeps people out of trouble and keeps society a little safer. However, in order to create more genuine and long-lasting change, going a little deeper is necessary. The next three tools will start you in this direction.

While core beliefs were addressed in Chapter 6, this tool identifies some common assumptions or conditional beliefs flowing from those core beliefs that give rise to your target behaviors. These are specifically common to people who deal with criminal thinking and rule-breaking behavior. Peruse the following checklist. Put an "X" by any of the intermediate beliefs that apply to you.

- ❏ "It is not my fault if I hurt someone else. If they get hurt, they deserve it"
- ❏ "I will always get away with it"
- ❏ "Everyone breaks rules—and—some people do a lot worse things than me"
- ❏ "It is okay to rob businesses. They have plenty of money and I need some excitement in my life"
- ❏ "My homeboys look after me. I am not like those straight-arrow people"
- ❏ "You'll never get justice from the legal system, so you have to get it yourself"
- ❏ "Even though I got caught once doesn't mean I'll get caught again. They got lucky"
- ❏ "Talking about feelings is for weaklings. If I open up, I'll get taken advantage of"

Now, use a thought log to challenge, dispute, or argue with each of those beliefs you checked. Use logic, advice from those on your team, past evidence, and anything else you want to, in an attempt to change your thinking in these areas.

My Thought Log

Automatic Thought	Rational Responses

Tool #14: Mode Messages

Practitioners of schema therapy have noted that people with PDs have some specific themes in their "states of being" that can include moods and behaviors that are distinct from the run-of-the-mill mood swings that all people have. They have called these state-like experiences schema *modes*. These can be triggered on a moment's notice, and specific modes have distinct characteristics. Certain constellations of beliefs and modes are associated with different PDs. The four modes associated with ASPD are called:

1. **Angry Protector Mode:** In this state, people experience intense anger, but it is controlled. They are able to use it as a "wall" to protect themselves.

2. **Predator Mode:** This is a state in which aggressive and even violent behaviors can be displayed in a very callous, cold, uncaring, and unempathetic manner. The purpose is often exacting revenge or eliminating a threat.

3. **Conning and Manipulative Mode:** This is a state many rule-breakers "flip" into in which they, often times in a premeditated and calculating way, plan and carry out manipulative or exploitive behaviors for personal profit or pleasure.

4. **Over-Controller Mode:** This is a place many people with ASPD find themselves in; it involves focusing one's attention on a person or entity that is perceived as threatening, seeking them out, and engaging in controlling behaviors in an attempt to either target them or to stay safe.

The message is different in each mode, but most, if not all, of these "parts" of you exist if you fall somewhere on the antisocial spectrum. Use this tool to describe specific behavior you have engaged in that you recognize as indicative of the above modes.

- Angry Protector Mode _____
  _____
  _____
  _____

- Predator Mode _____
  _____
  _____
  _____

- Conning and Manipulative Mode _____
  _____
  _____
  _____

- Over-Controller Mode _____
  _____
  _____
  _____

- The mode I most relate with _____

- One step I will take to work on these behaviors _____

Tool #15: Attachment

Attachment is a really important part of the developmental processes. Without healthy, secure attachments, it is next to impossible to connect with other humans in a meaningful way. It is very difficult for people with ASPD to genuinely connect with other people, including a therapist. Since connection is an important part of improving through treatment, it is one of the factors that makes work with this population challenging. If this is you, you know exactly what I am referring to. You may even take pride in your superficial charm which enables you to con and manipulate people, fuels a resistance to genuineness and authentic human connection, and keeps you from caring.

Connecting with others is a vital step of genuine growth. So, for those of you not just pretending to take this seriously, use the following tool to get yourself and your therapist started exploring attachment.

Attachment Tool

- To me, connecting with people means _____
  _____

- I know somebody wants to connect with me when _____
_____
_____

- I want to connect with somebody else when _____
_____
_____

- People I have genuinely connected with in the past are _____
_____
_____

- I know I can count on others to be there for me because _____
_____
_____

- Others can have faith I will be there for them because _____
_____
_____

- When I hurt somebody I feel _____
_____
_____

- Somebody deserves to be punished when _____
_____
_____

- I know somebody is worthy of me going to bat for them because _____
_____
_____

- When someone I care about gets hurt or killed due to an altercation which I instigated, I feel _____
_____
_____

- I feel I can connect with an animal better than a person because _____
_____
_____

- I can see some benefits of attaching to someone, like _____
_____
_____

CHAPTER 7:
THE NARCISSISTIC PERSONALITY DISORDER

The Narcissistic Personality Disorder

Hidden agenda: To achieve and to maintain special status

Prevalence rates: 1-6% of the general population

Gender distribution: More commonly diagnosed in men than women

Cognitive profile:

- View of self: "I am special"

- View of others: Most others are inferior ("There are a few other special people")

- View of world: "The world has two sets of 'rules'"

Common schemas: Spoiled entitlement, emotional deprivation, defectiveness, unrelenting standards, subjugation, approval seeking, insufficient self-control

Common cognitive distortions: Personalization, "should" statements (directed towards others), rationalization

Overdeveloped traits: Self-aggrandizement, competitiveness

Underdeveloped traits: Empathy, sharing

Whom they date/marry: Dependents, other narcissists

Where they work: Physicians, attorneys, TV/radio personalities, politicians, professional athletes

Other Random Nuggets:

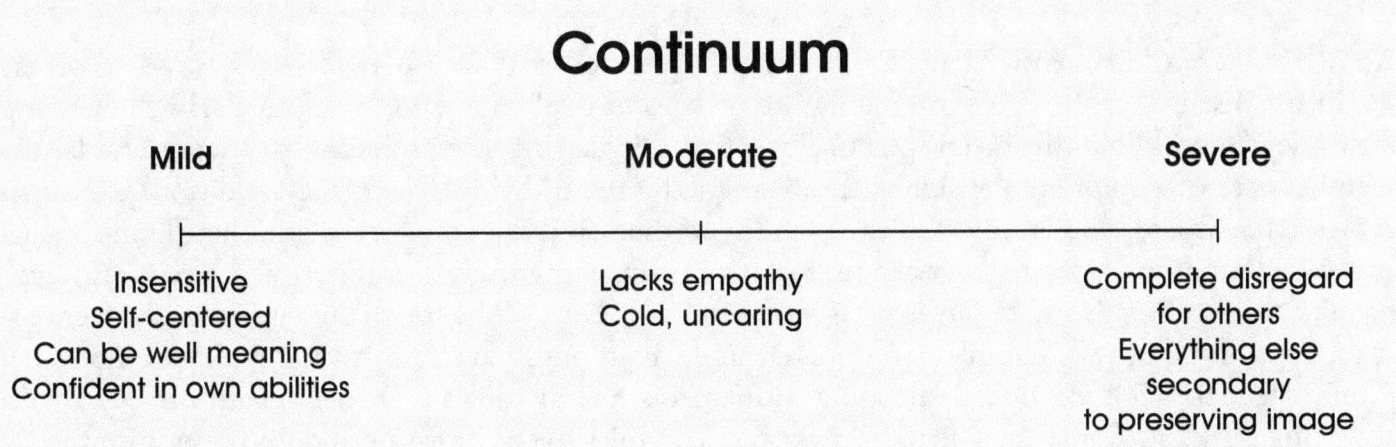

Tool #1: Trait Checklist

Individuals that suffer from the characteristics of narcissistic personality disorder (NPD) have a number of commonalities. Whether you are a loved one has this full blown condition, or some of the traits of it, survey the following checklist. The more of these you check yes to, the more likely it is this pattern of behavior is causing some problems occupationally, relationally, or socially.

- ❑ Believes they are in some way better than others

- ❑ Associates mainly with other "special" people

- ❑ Needs to be admired or looked up to by others

- ❑ Criticism and/or lack of recognition of perceived status produces intensely hurt feelings

- ❑ Can be overly focused on success, power, brilliance, or the perfect partner

- ❑ Marginalizes, minimizes, or devalues others behind their backs or talks in demeaning ways to their faces

- ❑ Expects special favors and gets angry if you don't give them "what they have a right to"

- ❑ Lacks empathy—has a very difficult time "putting themselves in someone else's shoes"

- ❑ Insists on having the best of everything — for instance, the best car or office

Tool #2: Expressions of Concern

All people have what are often called "blind spots": qualities we don't see in ourselves as well as others see in us. Because of the ego-syntonic nature of PDs, this phenomenon is particularly challenging for these people. What this means practically is that things that pose problems for friends and family members are often not are considered problematic by the individual with the condition. Concerns expressed by friends and family may have validity to them, but due to poor insight, the PD individual generally has difficulty seeing how certain behaviors impact themselves or others negatively. However, not all concerns friends and family express have validity. So, one of the tough but vital steps for recovery is sorting through these "complaints" to determine which ones have validity and which do not. One thing that makes this exercise challenging for narcissistic individuals is their inherent difficulty with accepting criticism. Some are able to hear concerns on the subject, however, and for them this exercise can be useful.

Use the following tool to identify *who* has expressed concern, *what* the exact concerns are, and *why* they see them as potentially hurtful. Look at the example, then complete your own and answer the questions that follow.

Person Expressing Concern	Action Causing Concern	Reason for Concern
1. Boss	1. Multiple complaints from coworkers	1. Office morale; "he doesn't want to have to fire me because I am the best worker"
2. Wife	2. Working long hours	2. Marital problems
3. Children at college	3. Potential affairs	3. Fears of family breaking up
4. Friend Joe	4. Smoking pot and occasionally other illegal drugs	4. Legal and health concerns

Questions:

- Who are three people I trust to "shoot straight" with me, by whom I can run these concerns to get their opinion?

    1. Joe

    2. ?

    3. ?

- With which concerns can I at least see where the person is coming from?

    Job concerns—I am the best person on that team by far, so he will never fire me

- Which concerns can I see the most validity in?

    Affair—I am having one, but nobody really knows about it. But it could break up our family

- I am willing to take the following steps to change one of the concerns:

    1. Keep going to therapy to talk about it

    2. ?

    3. ?

My Expressions of Concern

Person Expressing Concern	Action Causing Concern	Reason for Concern
1.	1.	1.
2.	2.	2.
3.	3.	3.
4.	4.	4.
5.	5.	5.

Questions:

- Who are three people I trust to "shoot straight" with me, by whom I can run these concerns by to get their opinion?

    1. _____

    2. _____

    3. _____

- With which concerns can I at least see where the person is coming from? _____
  _____
  _____

- Which concerns can I see the most validity in? _____
  _____
  _____

- I am willing to take the following steps to change one of the concerns
  1. _____
  2. _____
  3. _____

Tool #3: Pros and Cons

This tool helps you evaluate the potential pros and cons of your narcissistic behaviors. It is called a *four-box pros and cons*. Sometimes it can be beneficial to look at not only the advantages and disadvantages of maintaining certain behaviors but also the advantages and disadvantages of changing them. After listing the pros and cons of each, it can be even more helpful to rate, on a scale of 0-10, how important each item is. Consider the example that is provided. Then complete one on your own!

Example: Pros and Cons of Avoiding Behavior

Pros of Remaining Unempathetic	Pros of Developing Some Empathy
I win at any cost (8)	Better marriage with my wife (8)
Will always be success (10)	My daughter might spend more time with me (10)
Don't have to waste time (7)	Employees like me better (7)

Cons of Remaining Unempathetic	Cons of Developing Some Empathy
I upset my wife (8)	I would have to care what other people feel (6)
Create tension with employees (3)	Would be less productive (6)
Daughter doesn't like me very much (10)	

Results:

__25__ Reasons to remain unempathetic

__21__ Reasons to not remain unempathetic

__25__ Reasons to work on empathy

__12__ Reasons to not gain empathy

My Conclusions: These traits have motivated me and served me well professionally, but I am starting to pay for it on the home front

My Commitment:

1. I will cut back to 60 hours/week

2. I will plan one outing with my daughter each month

Analysis: This is a client in his upper fifties who has spent a great deal of his life running over people. He is finally to the point where his relationships are starting to matter at least a little to him, as he has begun to realize some of the damage that he has done. Because of this, I am convinced that if I encountered him, say, ten years ago, his prognosis would be much more guarded that it was when I actually met him. It is typical that he is much more bothered by the prospect of his employees "not liking him" than he is by the "tension" between them. Also, his relationship with his daughter seems more meaningful than that with his wife, so this leverage will be utilized moving forward in treatment.

My Pros and Cons of Low-Empathy Behavior

Pros of Remaining Unempathetic	Pros of Developing Some Empathy
Cons of Remaining Unempathetic	**Cons of Developing Some Empathy**

Results:

_____ Reasons to remain unempathetic

_____ Reasons to not remain unempathetic

_____ Reasons to gain empathy

_____ Reasons to not gain empathy

My Conclusions _____
_____
_____
_____

My Commitment(s) _____
_____
_____
_____
_____

Tool #4: Identify Behavioral Targets

Although low empathy is a theme in narcissism, this trait can manifest differently in different people. Some behaviors include demeaning or ignoring others, name calling, and taking about others in a belittling way. People with low empathy often become indignant when somebody doesn't recognize their status. They can 1) become rageful or 2) feel deeply hurt when not recognized. Running over others is a frequent occurrence. "Name dropping," resumé reciting, or pointing out that they own the finest things in life can also be attempts to help others notice their "specialness."

Use this tool to identify some of your narcissistic behaviors that you or others have noticed. Feel free to use any of the above behaviors that fit, or list some of your own.

- **Behaviors related to my low empathy traits that I or someone else identified which I am willing to target to improve my situation:**

    1. _____
    2. _____
    3. _____
    4. _____
    5. _____

Tool #5: Intimacy Circles

Intimacy is a scary word for a lot of people. If the sound of it makes you cringe, this exercise is definitely for you—and even if it doesn't, this exercise likely will still benefit you. It will benefit almost everyone in some way. Why? Because almost everyone could benefit from improving at least one interpersonal relationship in their life. Some people's lives could be enriched with more friends. Others need to learn to set boundaries with someone in their life. A lot of people have "trust issues." Yet others would be happier in life if they learned to pick healthier people to date or form friendships with; toxic people have a way of draining people of their energy and joy. A certain percentage of the population would be much less prone to mood swings if they could be okay alone. Some would find more fulfillment in life if they could share more with people in their lives; others would not be hurt as often if they learned to share less with those in their life. A lot of people walk around with their "walls" up. Some have difficulty expressing feelings. Some have been accused of being too "needy." Others have difficulty asking for help.

You may have heard intimacy defined as "Into-Me-See"—the degree to which we let people see into us, and vice versa. A lot of my clients have found this "play on words" to be a helpful way to remember its definition and connotations.

Use the following tool to evaluate the relationships in your life. Use the percentage signs to help you decide which people to put in which circles. No other person goes in the ME circle (though some people choose to put God here). This is for you alone. People who belong in circle #1 are those with whom you would feel comfortable sharing ANY problem in life, no matter how personal (a sexual problem, something related to an abusive situation, a salary issue, etc.). People in circle #2 are those in your life with whom there may be a personal issue or two (like the ones mentioned above) that you would not share, but you would be comfortable sharing ALMOST anything (roughly 75%) about your life. People in circle #3 may get about half of your personal stuff, but the other half you probably would not trust them with. People in circle #4 would be your very casual relationships. Maybe they know whether you are married or where you work or something of that nature, but you don't share very much with them (roughly 25%). And people in circle #5 get nothing. For some people, these are individuals whom they have just met, so they could be candidates to move closer in as they get to know them. Or, these are people who at one point in life were closer in, but they have done something to violate trust, so they have had to be moved out one or more rings.

If you are a person with low empathy, it is likely people don't like you. Sorry—just shooting straight with you. (Actually, I'm not sorry, since people who can't be direct do you no good. If you were blind folded and about to walk off a cliff, wouldn't you want someone to tell you?) Likely, your response to people not liking you is, "Their loss." And it may be. But remember, nobody is watching. Be honest about how much you really care about the people in your life. Although many people with narcissistic tendencies get defensive at these suggestions, it is those who are mature enough to consider something that doesn't initially feel good who are able to make meaningful changes. For most people with NPD, it starts with a willingness to be honest and genuine with just one person.

Keep these ideas in mind as you consider who truly belongs where as you complete your circles. Your first task is to think about all the people in your life and where they go in your circles. Then consider the questions that follow to get you started making healthy changes to your relationships. Work with your therapist or other helping professional if you need ongoing guidance or accountability.

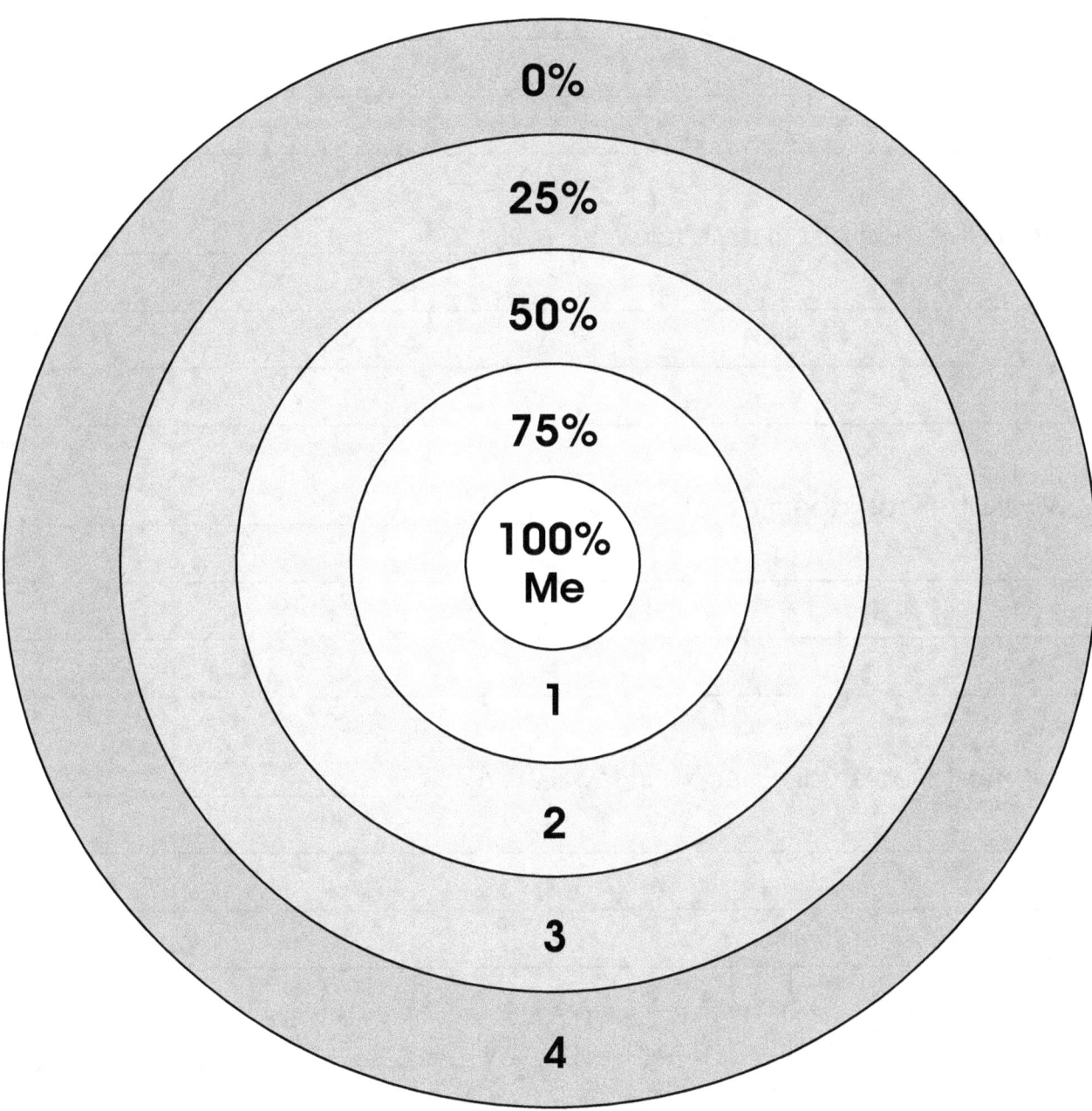

Intimacy Circles Follow-Up Starter Questions

- General observations about my circles _____
  _____
  _____
  _____

- What I like most about my circles _____
  _____
  _____
  _____

- What I like least about my circles _____
  _____
  _____
  _____

- The most problematic people in my life _____
  _____
  _____
  _____

- They are problematic in the following ways _____
  _____
  _____
  _____

- People in my life whose opinions I actually care about and on a scale of 0-10 how much I care what they think _____

_____

_____

_____

- People in my life whose opinions I have not been as concerned with as perhaps I should have been _____

_____

_____

- People in my life whom I have hurt due to arrogance, dismissiveness or insensitivity

_____

_____

_____

- People in my life who have moved themselves out in my circles due to my behavior

_____

_____

_____

- I could improve my circles if I were willing to treat the following people differently

_____

_____

_____

- One step I will take TODAY to treat people in my circles differently _____

_____

_____

Tool #6: Identify and Restructure Automatic Thoughts

A staple component of treatment for any psychological condition is recognizing the thought processes that are driving the problem behaviors and maintaining the symptoms. In colloquial language, you may hear this referred to as "self-talk." To speak in the terms of the Mark Twain quote in the introduction ("If all you have is a hammer, everything looks like a nail"): This is the "hammer." While treatment of personality disorders requires more tools than just a hammer, the hammer is still a useful tool to have in your toolbox.

Some people develop an awareness of their thoughts and get better at noticing them, but do nothing to change them. For example, if we recognize that we are overweight, but do nothing to change our diets or exercise levels, we will stay overweight. In the same way, if we recognize thoughts that are driving problem behavior but do nothing to change them, our symptoms are likely to remain.

So, one cognitive tool you can use is what is called challenging distorted thoughts when you recognize them. Refer to the beginning of this chapter for some distorted thoughts common in narcissistic personality disorder. *"Challenging,"* in this case, basically means "arguing" with the specific content of the thoughts. There are a number of techniques that can be used for doing this, including looking at evidence, seeking input from others, researching the facts, considering past or possible future results, or good old-fashioned logic, just to name a few.

The following tool asks you to identify specific low-empathy thoughts that enter your mind, challenge them in some way, and if you want to, rate your challenge on a scale of 0-10, indicating how meaningful the challenge is. Take a look at the example, and then do one on your own. This may be a tool that you will benefit from using on an ongoing basis.

Example: Thought Log

Low-Empathy Thought	Rational Responses
Since I am one of the most important people in this industry, people at this conference should recognize me and acknowledge my achievements	Maybe he didn't acknowledge me because he was intimidated (7) Maybe he is brand new to the industry, so that's why he didn't know who I was (8) Maybe he knew who I was, but has just been told not to be too friendly to competitors (7) Maybe he's just an idiot (10) Even though most people know who I am, a few people may not (5)

Analysis: Here we see typical attempts at rational responses from narcissists, particularly early in treatment. The challenges with the highest believability ratings all feed his "special" belief. He did rate the last one, which challenges that notion a bit, as a 5, so that is something, at least.

My Narcissistic Thought Log

Low-Empathy Thoughts	Rational Responses

Tool #7: Historical Experiences Worksheet

As with most, if not all, personality disorders, there are multiple pathways to NPD. Although it is known that NPD has at least a mild genetic component, this condition is believed to be developed largely due to environmental factors. Many people with these traits have some commonalities in their backgrounds of experience. Peruse the following historical experiences worksheet and put an "X" beside factors that were a part of your experiences from a young age.

- ❏ History of being lonely as a child
- ❏ History of being manipulated as a child
- ❏ History that involved conditional approval
- ❏ Parents rarely showed affection
- ❏ Parents had unrealistically high standards
- ❏ Surface-level conversation was rewarded
- ❏ Performance was emphasized
- ❏ "Ordinary" people were devalued
- ❏ Parents or caretakers failed set limits

- Describe how the experiences checked above apply specifically to you and the impact you believe they continue to have in your life today

_____
_____
_____
_____
_____
_____
_____
_____

Tool #8: Belief Identification

As has been discussed, all behaviors are a product of beliefs. Beliefs drive behavior. Due to the compelling nature of beliefs in individuals with PDs, these deeper-level beliefs often have to be modified to help create lasting change. As noted at the beginning of this chapter, common beliefs in people with NPD include spoiled entitlement, emotional deprivation, defectiveness, unrelenting standards, subjugation, approval seeking, and insufficient self-control. Review their definitions if you don't have them fresh in your mind. Get with your therapist. Include friends and family who are willing to give you feedback. Identify one or two beliefs that you believe drive your target behaviors to work on in treatment. Write them inside Judy Beck's "Pac-Man" visual aid (which was explained in the introduction).

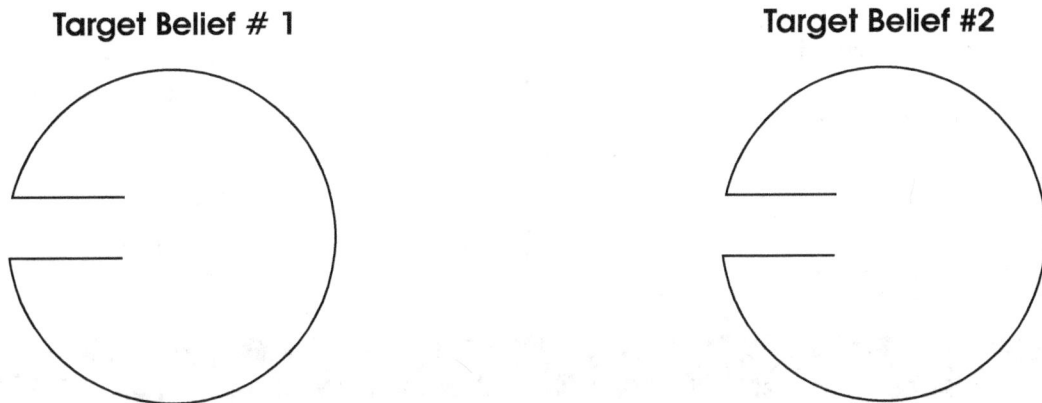

Beliefs always come in pairs. For every maladaptive (or unhealthy) belief we possess, we also possess an alternate, adaptive (or healthy) belief. For instance, even though an individual may have the belief, "I must be the one in charge," they also have the belief, however faint "Control is overrated."

I have given you the "pushing buttons" language, the "Pac-Man" visual, and the "filters" imagery. Here is another representation which I hope helps illustrate the point: We could think of beliefs as lenses. For people who wear glasses, this visual probably comes fairly intuitively. Healthier individuals are able to engage in more balanced information processing. Figuratively speaking they are able to see out of both the left and the right "lenses" equally. This is the goal of belief modification work: balanced information processing. In other words, to be able to see both sides objectively and to be able to recognize when they fail or make mistakes, so they can learn from them; and also to be able to acknowledge when they succeed and be able to take a compliment. Although nobody is perfect and everyone has their biases, healthier people's lenses are closer to the 50/50 range (50% failure/50% success). Before treatment, people with PDs, due to their more compelling beliefs, often start with numbers such as 99%/1%. **Intentional and sustained effort** is required to create a healthier belief balance.

So, now that you have identified your unhealthy beliefs driving your target behaviors, identify in your own words what you would call the opposite, healthy belief. Write it in the opposite belief structure that the "triangle" could fit into.

After you have identified your one or two healthy and unhealthy beliefs, ask yourself: "What percentage of the time do I believe the unhealthy belief? What percentage of the time do I believe the healthy belief?" Write your numbers in the line next to each belief (they should total 100%). Then you are ready to move on to Tool #9!

See the example first, and then do one on your own!

Example: Belief Identification

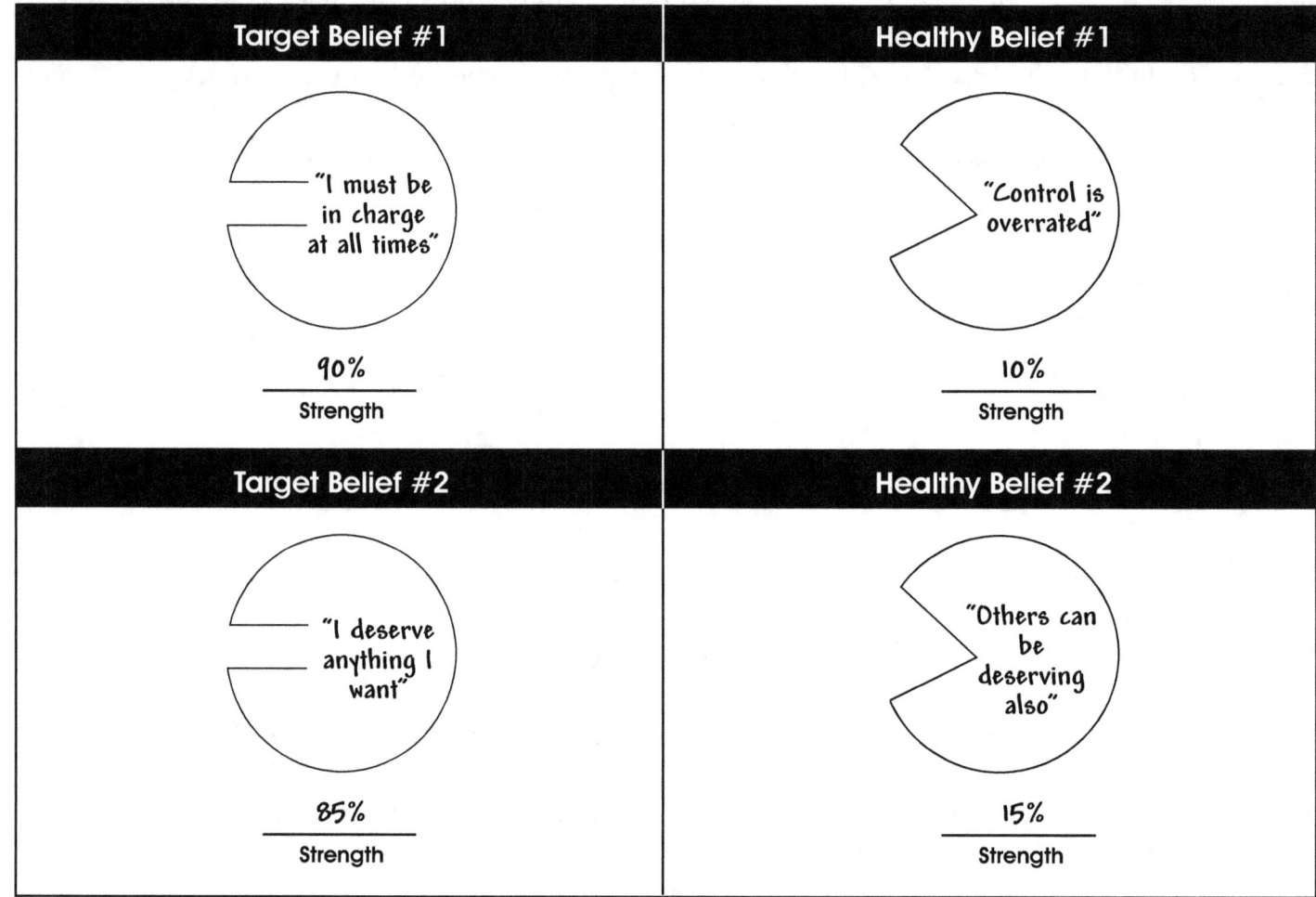

My Beliefs

Target Belief #1	Healthy Belief #1
Strength	Strength
Target Belief #2	**Healthy Belief #2**
Strength	Strength

Tool #9: Evidence Logs

Here is where the hard work begins! This is a tool you will use throughout your treatment, regardless of what other tools you may be using and at what stage of treatment you may be at. This is the tough, tough work of gradually working to develop your healthy belief. How do we change beliefs, anyway? It's a difficult process, no doubt. What we need to do is to *reexamine historical evidence, get better at noticing current evidence* **and** *intentionality initiate ongoing experiences around which to create new evidence.*

Think of any belief that you have changed over time in any area of your life. Maybe you used to not believe in God and now you do. Perhaps you used to not believe in global warming and now you do. Maybe you used to believe in life on other planets and now you don't. For example, I have a client who is a marine biology major in college – his chief interest is in Megalodon sharks, which he was initially convinced were not extinct. After a lot of scientific research, he now no longer believes that. Did you used to hold more conservative political beliefs, and your beliefs are now more progressive? You get the gist. You can use a belief that you have changed in *any* area of life to illustrate this process. How do

beliefs change? By examining the evidence created by experience and the meaning that we assign to it.

Take a belief many people once held. (WARNING! UPCOMING CONTENT NOT APPROPRIATE FOR KIDS!) Santa Claus is not real. If you believed in his existence when you were six years old, what was the "evidence" that supported your belief? He brought presents. They said "from Santa" on the wrapping. He drank the milk that was set out for him. He knew what presents were desired from the letters that was sent to him at the North Pole. The local weather even tracks him on the Doppler radar!

Over time, most people reexamine the pieces of evidence and assign new meaning to them. By doing so, they change their belief.

But they have to *experience* new evidence.

Some children recognize Papa beneath the Santa suit and false white beard. Some children stay up all night and sneak downstairs to catch a parent putting presents under the tree. Some children are observant enough to notice that "Santa" has Mommy's identical hand writing or wrapping paper. The child who *does not go out of their way to look for these things* holds onto the old, false belief much longer because they are not looking for evidence to the contrary. In fact, when I myself was becoming suspicious but desperately wanted to believe that he was real as a child, I began actively searching out confirmation of his existence.

In the same way, for any of us to change our beliefs, we must be *willing* to examine evidence fairly. We are naturally (consciously or unconsciously) looking for evidence to support our existing belief. But we must be equally willing to consider evidence to the contrary as well. This is what the evidence logs do: they provide a tool to facilitate *purposefully looking for evidence* to support the new belief you are attempting to construct. If your current unhealthy belief is that you are a failure, then you are purposefully looking for evidence that you can succeed. For some cognitive behavioral therapy (CBT) exercises, we will ask people to log evidence on *both* sides. But because people with PDs have such deeply engrained beliefs, their natural tendency will be to see only evidence that supports the current belief. So, for the purpose of this exercise, it is important to use the right column only to log evidence that supports the belief. The left column will remain blank.

As you record the evidence, think about how it felt to have that experience. As you do, ask yourself: *In this moment* how much do I believe _____ and how much do I believe _____?
                                                 (unhealthy belief)   (healthy belief)

Remember, you will inherently *not notice* evidence that will be helpful because your filter is directing you away from it, so be vigilant. Also, when you log evidence for a healthy belief, you will get that little voice in your head that says, "but… it doesn't count because of this or that." Go ahead and record the evidence anyway even if you have trouble believing it at the time.

Log the believability rating as you record each piece of evidence. Note that these numbers will go up

and down, because beliefs fluctuate. But over time, watch your unhealthy numbers generally trend down and your healthy numbers trend up. The more they change, the more balanced your lenses will be come and you will get your "buttons pushed" less frequently!

Look at the example below. Then begin completing your own evidence log, working on one belief at a time. When you have more than one icebergs to conquer, the more effort you put into chiseling one at a time, the more progress you will make.

Example: Evidence Log

Date	Unhealthy Belief: 90% "I must be in charge at all times"	% Belief	Healthy Belief: 10% "Control is overrated"	% Belief
12/2		75%	Chose not to yell at employee when screwed up – felt good about it	25%
12/9		80%	Let wife make decision about restaurant	20%
12/12		80%	Didn't interrupt Joe and reprimand him in the meeting	20%
12/19		80%	Was patient with the waitress when she didn't do what I told her to do	20%
12/22		75%	Let somebody else decide the order of songs we practiced at the Christmas ensemble	25%

Conclusions: I have been less in control and done allright, but I don't see too much harm being done by being totally in control

My Evidence Log

Unhealthy Belief: _____   **Healthy Belief:** _____

Date		% Belief		% Belief

Conclusion: _____
_____

Tool #10: Protect Your Image!

Andre Agassi, in addition to being one of the top ten tennis players of all time, was famous for the commercial in which he said, "Image is everything!" As someone who grew up in the Agassi era (as well as played college tennis wearing similar denims and spandex), it shocked me to read his autobiography years later and discover what was behind the image. I am not saying Agassi was a narcissist; but what I saw when the curtain was pulled back was certainly revealing to me and, to many, down right shocking.

Similarly, the image the narcissist usually projects portrays an existence that is drastically different from what one would see if the curtain were pulled back. If you are reading this as someone who has NPD, you know exactly what I am talking about (although you may not show it to anyone very often). All people, narcissistic or not, protect their image to one degree or another. There is actually a thing called "healthy narcissism." It is the extreme versions of this, however, that creates problems in people with narcissistic traits. Think about ways in which your narcissism has hurt you. Perhaps revisit your circles in Tool #5 or your pros and cons in Tool #3. Now utilize the following tool to think about some ways you can protect your image that would not create unwanted consequences.

"Image is Everything!" Tool

- Some ways I can maintain my image without the damaging consequences I have experienced in the past

    1. _____
    2. _____
    3. _____
    4. _____
    5. _____

Tool #11: Mode Messages

Practitioners of schema therapy have noted that people with PDs have some specific themes in their "states of being" that can include moods and behaviors that are distinct from the run-of-the-mill mood swings that all people have. They have called these state-like experiences schema *modes*. These can be triggered on a moment's notice, and specific modes have distinct characteristics. Certain constellations of beliefs and modes are associated with different PDs. The four modes associated with NPD are called:

1. **Lonely Child Mode:** This mode manifests in terms of feelings of loneliness, emptiness, or inferiority. Some people with NPD are not self-aware enough to be in touch with these feelings, but if you have this PD, this is the mode you need to be capable of "going to" in order to make the most meaningful improvement. A skilled therapist may facilitate your staying in this mode by imagery, inclusion of invested significant others, or other therapeutic techniques. It has been hypothesized that not all people with NPD have this mode. If this is the case, prognosis for these individuals is likely much worse.

2. **Enraged Child Mode:** This mode is triggered by the inability to tolerate intense painful feelings, usually triggered by a criticism of some kind. Flipping into enraged child mode usually guarantees problematic consequences from a spouse, employer, or other person with whom you interact on a regular basis.

3. **Detached Self-Soother:** This mode is flipped into when a narcissistic individual cannot bear their feelings of defectiveness and must detach from those feelings. This mode often involves use of alcohol, drugs, or engaging in sexual or other addictive behavior with the motivation of self-soothing.

4. **Self-Aggrandizer Mode:** This is the mode individuals with NPD are most noted for. This manifests in belittling, demeaning, yelling, arrogance, dismissive responses, controlling behavior, and many other actions that likely have been identified by you or someone else as target behaviors. If this is you, know that as long as you stay in this mode, it is next to impossible to get better.

The message is different in each mode, but most, if not all of these "parts" of you exist if you fall somewhere on the NPD spectrum. Use this tool to describe specific behavior you have engaged in that you recognize as part of the above modes.

- Lonely Child Mode _____
_____
_____
_____

- Enraged Child Mode _____
  _____
  _____
  _____

- Detached Self-Soother Mode _____
  _____
  _____
  _____

- Self- Aggrandizer Mode _____
  _____
  _____
  _____

- The mode I most relate with _____

- One step I will take to work on these behaviors _____

Tool #12: Lowering the Bar

Although it is not considered a "core belief," one of the compensatory schemas associated with NPD, as noted at the beginning of this chapter, is a version of the "unrelenting standards" belief. People with OCPD and other perfectionistic individuals also have a version of this schema. While narcissists can be perfectionistic, they usually don't require those behaviors of others or get angry with them when they fail to meet their high standards; in fact, if you have narcissistic traits, you don't expect most others to meet your high standards or complete great achievements because you don't view them as capable of it. Only "special" people are capable of achieving "special" status. The individual with NPD holds these high standards only for themselves. This belief drives them to outwork other people and often helps them soar to supervisory roles and gives them a seat beside the privileged of society. Achieving these standards is the primary supporting evidence for their belief that they are special. Entitlement- related cognitions, are most prominent in self-aggrandizing mode. This might even manifest in smaller ways, such as always flying first class (and taking extreme pride in your gold elite status), requiring the highest quality coffee, or always paying for the high-end suites at the local sporting event or performing arts venue.

One small step people with narcissistic tendencies can take is to identify areas of life where you have sought these highest standards and look for small ways you could modify them in order to "lower the bar" at least a bit. The goal is to learn that it is possible to modify your standards, yet still be excellent.

High-Standard Behavior	Small Ways I Could Modify Standards
1.	
2.	
3.	

Tool #13: Valuing Others

Individuals with borderline personality disorder are known for flipping between idealizing others to devaluing others; people with NPD, on the other hand, just devalue others. Devaluing cognitively (seeing them as "all bad," "completely inferior," or "not in my league") is what leads to the behaviors exhibited in self-aggrandizer mode. It also contributes to the lack of empathy (one of the other diagnostic criteria). Before one can empathize, they must be able to see some value in the other person. This is not an easy process for someone with NPD. Remember, even those who try will have to deal with immediate discounting thoughts and the resulting defensive reactions. So this won't come for you overnight. But this tool is designed to help you see some value in others.

- The person I am working to see some value in _____

- Some qualities I currently see as valuable in others _____

_____
_____

- Does this person have any of these qualities to any degree? If so, which qualities?
  _____
  _____
  _____

- Now consider qualities that person has on which you have historically *not* placed high value. List these positive qualities you see in them _____
  _____
  _____

- Pick one quality that you listed above which you can see at least see some value in, even if it hasn't been overly important or impressive to you _____
  _____
  _____

- Why did you pick that quality? What is it about that characteristic that enables you to see it in a positive light to some degree? _____
  _____
  _____

- Describe a specific situation in which you saw the person exhibit that quality. What was the situation? What specifically did they do that you respected?
  _____
  _____
  _____

When your "autopilot" thoughts are inclined to devalue this person, remind yourself of why they are important to you and what you have to lose if you act on those thoughts.

- I am working to respect this person because
  1. _____
  2. _____
  3. _____

Tool #14: Building Empathy

One hallmark of individuals with NPD is the lack of empathy. You have even heard narcissistic individuals characterized in this book as "low-empathy" individuals.

Empathy can be defined as *the ability to understand and share the feelings of another person*. Putting yourself in another person's shoes can be difficult. Use this tool to attempt to develop some empathy for someone in your life.

- Who is the person in my life it would benefit me to empathize with? _____

- It is difficult for me to empathize with them because _____
  _____
  _____

- My guess is someone in their position might be thinking _____
  _____
  _____

- Their goal in this situation is _____
  _____
  _____

- The people in their life they have to be accountable to are _____
  _____
  _____

- If I were in their position, I would probably feel _____
  _____
  _____

- Describe the position they are in from their perspective _____
_____
_____

- I was in a similar position when _____
_____
_____

- Even though I have never been in that exact position, I know what it feels like to
_____
_____
_____

- Based upon my empathizing with them, it would be more effective for me to cope in the following different ways _____
_____
_____

- Behaviors which I or someone else identified and which I am willing to target in order to improve my situation

    1. _____
    2. _____
    3. _____
    4. _____
    5. _____

Tool #15: Go Deep!

As a football fan, I had to name a tool "Go Deep!" As I stated with a previous tool, there almost shouldn't be a tool for this one—but this is a toolbox, after all, and narcissistic (as well as histrionic) individuals have difficulty with this issue. The application of this tool can be difficult and requires consistent work over time, not to mention a willingness to 1) share the attention in the dialogue as well as 2) "go deep," which does not come natural for you if you have this particular set of personality traits. It simply involves building an authentic relationship with someone—hopefully, eventually, more than one someone. But we all have to start somewhere. Use this tool to facilitate the process for yourself.

- The person in my life I am willing to try to "go deep" with _____

- I commit to meet with them _____
  (how often)

- I have known that person for _____
  (length of time)

- I know the following things about them _____
  _____
  _____

- To my knowledge, they know the following things about me _____
  _____
  _____

- I commit to share one thing per week with them which I have not shared with anyone previously, going from least personal to most personal over time. I also agree to express my needs to them over time. Some personal information I will share as our relationship deepens _____
  _____
  _____

- I commit to being cognizant of time and allowing them to share with me as well. I will monitor my responses and attempt to be supportive. If they share some constructive criticism, I will make every attempt to receive it, even if I feel myself getting defensive.

- Some things I look forward to learning about them _____
_____
_____

- Some questions I will ask them _____
_____
_____

- Some areas in which they may confront me that may be uncomfortable to me
_____
_____
_____

- Some values we have in common that we can discuss _____
_____
_____

- Some hobbies we have in common that we can discuss _____
_____
_____

- When I am tempted to cancel a meeting or walk away from the relationship, here are some things I can remind myself of _____
_____
_____

- Questions or comments I have for my therapist as I embark on this journey _____
_____
_____
_____

Chapter 7: The Narcissistic Personality Disorder

CHAPTER 8: THE PARANOID PERSONALITY DISORDER

The Paranoid Personality Disorder

Hidden agenda: To stay safe

Prevalence rates: 2-4% of the general population

Gender distribution: More common in men than women

Cognitive profile:

- View of self: "I am vulnerable"
- View of others: "Others are out to get me"
- View of world: "The world is dangerous"

Common schemas: Mistrust, vulnerability, punitiveness

Common cognitive distortions: Personalization, mind reading, fortune telling, "should" statements (directed towards others)

Overdeveloped traits: Vigilance, suspiciousness

Underdeveloped traits: Trust, acceptance

Whom they date/marry: Nobody

Where they work: Often unemployed

Other Random Nuggets: Higher levels of violence than many people realize

Continuum

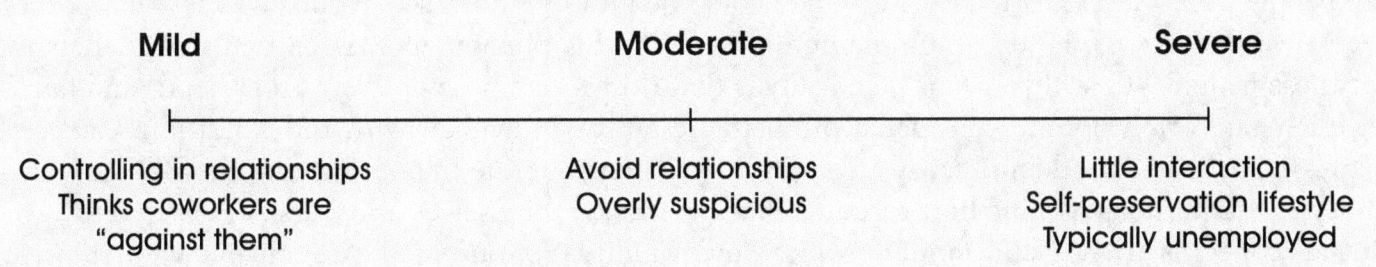

Tool #1: Trait Checklist

Individuals that suffer from the characteristics of paranoid personality disorder (PPD) have a number of commonalities. Whether you are a loved one has this full blown condition, or some of the traits of it, survey the following checklist. The more of these you check yes to, the more likely it is this pattern of behavior is causing some problems occupationally, relationally, or socially.

- ☐ Thinks everyone is out to get them
- ☐ Can't trust anyone
- ☐ Withholds personal information for fear it will be used against them
- ☐ Takes comments which others would not think anything of as personal attacks
- ☐ Finds it almost impossible to forgive others
- ☐ Has difficulty seeing their role in interpersonal problems (it is always the other's fault)
- ☐ Feels intense anger when slighted
- ☐ Strongly dislikes accountability
- ☐ Often times not in romantic relationships
- ☐ Constantly suspects infidelity in relationships with no evidence
- ☐ Oftentimes works "on the side," choosing to have no official employer
- ☐ Misinterprets non-threatening situations to be threatening

Tool #2: Expressions of Concern

All people have what are often called "blind spots": qualities we don't see in ourselves as well as others see in us. Because of the ego-syntonic nature of PDs, this phenomenon is particularly challenging for these people. What this means practically is that things that pose problems for friends and family members are often not are considered problematic by the individual with the condition. Concerns expressed by friends and family may have validity to them, but due to poor insight, the PD individual generally has difficulty seeing how certain behaviors impact themselves or others negatively. However, not all concerns friends and family express have validity. So, one of the tough but vital steps for recovery is sorting through these "complaints" to determine which ones have validity and which do not. Obviously, the biggest problem for people with paranoia is that when you don't trust anyone, it is difficult to give validity to anyone's feedback.

Use the following tool to identify *who* has expressed concern, *what* the exact concerns are, and *why* they see them as potentially hurtful. Look at the example, then complete your own and answer the questions that follow.

Example:

Person Expressing Concern	Action Causing Concern	Reason for Concern
1. Mom	1. Don't leave the house enough	1. Thinks I'll get depressed
2. Therapist	2.	2.
3. ?	3.	3.

Questions:

- Who are three people I trust to "shoot straight" with me, by whom I can run these concerns to get their opinion?

    1. Therapist

    2. Mom

    3. ?

- With which concerns can I at least see where the person is coming from?

    She doesn't realize what a dangerous world it is

- Which concerns can I see the most validity in?

    I am lonely

- I am willing to take the following steps to change one of the concerns
    1. Keep going to therapy
    2. Go out and sit in the park for thirty minutes sometimes
    3. Go to church with my mom

My Expressions of Concern

Person Expressing Concern	Action Causing Concern	Reason for Concern
1.	1.	1.
2.	2.	2.
3.	3.	3.
4.	4.	4.
5.	5.	5.

Questions:

- Who are three people I trust to "shoot straight" with me, by whom I can run these concerns by to get their opinion?

    1. _____

    2. _____

    3. _____

- With which concerns can I at least see where the person is coming from? _____
  _____
  _____

- Which concerns can I see the most validity in? _____
  _____
  _____

- I am willing to take the following steps to change one of the concerns
    1. _____
    2. _____
    3. _____

Tool #3: Pros and Cons

This tool helps you evaluate the potential pros and cons of your paranoia behaviors. It is called a *four-box pros and cons*. Sometimes it can be beneficial to look at not only the advantages and disadvantages of maintaining certain behaviors but also the advantages and disadvantages of changing them. After listing the pros and cons of each, it can be even more helpful to rate on a scale of 0-10 how important each item is. Consider the example that is provided. Then complete one on your own!

Example: Pros and Cons of Suspicious Behavior

Pros of Remaining Suspicious	Pros of Developing Some Ability to Trust
Stay safe (9)	Won't be so anxious (7)
Stay in control (8)	Could have a friend (7)
	Wouldn't be so lonely (9)

Cons of Remaining Suspicious	Cons of Developing Some Ability to Trust
Stay anxious (8)	Could get hurt physically (6)
No friends (8)	Could get embarrassed (8)
Stay depressed (8)	Could get arrested (4)
	Could get exposed (9)

Results:

__17__ Reasons to remain suspicious

__24__ Reasons to not remain suspicious

__23__ Reasons to develop trust

__27__ Reasons to not develop trust

My Conclusions: I don't want to be so lonely; I just can't get it out of my head that people want to hurt me

My Commitment:

1. Go spend some time with my friend Ted this week
2. Go to church with my mom

Analysis: In this case, the client still has more reasons against rather than for trusting, although the numbers were closer than he thought they might have been. He clearly has extremely compelling mistrust related beliefs, but he has some motivation not to life the rest of his life lonely. Treatment will focus on developing trust for the purpose of developing some ability to have a friend or two whom he can at least somewhat trust.

My Pros and Cons of Suspicious Behavior

Pros of Remaining Suspicious	Pros of Developing Some Ability to Trust
Cons of Remaining Suspicious	**Cons of Developing Some Ability to Trust**

Results:

_____ Reasons to remain suspicious

_____ Reasons to not remain suspicious

_____ Reasons to develop trust

_____ Reasons to not develop trust

My Conclusions _____

_____

_____

My Commitment(s) _____

_____

_____

_____

_____

Tool #4: Identify Behavioral Targets

Paranoia manifests differently in different people. Some people have milder versions and some more severe. Some common behaviors include not leaving the house, avoiding employment, becoming quick to anger, making accusations, being unwilling to forgive, following others to make sure they are not following you, and using recording devices or other technology to collect "evidence."

Use this tool to identify some of your suspicious behaviors that you or others have noticed. Feel free to use any of the above behaviors that fit, or list some of your own.

- **Behaviors related to my paranoid traits that I or someone else identified which I am willing to target to improve my situation**

    1. _____
    2. _____
    3. _____
    4. _____
    5. _____

Tool #5: Intimacy Circles

Intimacy is a scary word for a lot of people. If the sound of it makes you cringe, this exercise is definitely for you—and even if it doesn't, this exercise likely will still benefit you. It will benefit almost everyone in some way. Why? Because almost everyone could benefit from improving at least one interpersonal relationship in their life. Some people's lives could be enriched with more friends. Others need to learn to set boundaries with someone in their life. A lot of people have "trust issues." Yet others would be happier in life if they learned to pick healthier people to date or form friendships with; toxic people have a way of draining people of their energy and joy. A certain percentage of the population would be much less prone to mood swings if they could be okay alone. Some would find more fulfillment in life if they could share more with people in their lives; others would not be hurt as often if they learned to share less with those in their life. A lot of people walk around with their "walls" up. Some have difficulty expressing feelings. Some have been accused of being too "needy." Others have difficulty asking for help.

You may have heard intimacy defined as "Into-Me-See"——the degree to which we let people see into us, and vice versa. A lot of my clients have found this "play on words" to be a helpful way to remember its definition and connotations.

Use the following tool to evaluate the relationships in your life. Use the percentage signs to help you decide which people to put in which circles. No other person goes in the ME circle (though some people choose to put God here). This is for you alone. People who belong in circle #1 are those with whom you would feel comfortable sharing ANY problem in life, no matter how personal (a sexual problem, something related to an abusive situation, a salary issue, etc.). People in circle #2 are those in your life with whom there may be a personal issue or two (like the ones mentioned above) that you would not share, but you would be comfortable sharing ALMOST anything (roughly 75%) about your life. People in circle #3 may get about half of your personal stuff, but the other half you probably would not trust them with. People in circle #4 would be your very casual relationships. Maybe they know whether you are married or where you work or something of that nature, but you don't share very much with them (roughly 25%). And people in circle #5 get nothing. For some people, these are individuals whom they have just met, so they could be candidates to move closer in as they get to know them. Or, these are people who at one point in life were closer in, but they have done something to violate trust, so they have had to be moved out one or more rings.

If you have suspicious tendencies, you will likely have a visceral reaction to the prospect of "letting people in." You probably experienced a bout of irritable bowel syndrome when you just read the word "intimacy." Although every bone in your body will want to resist this, if you have decided there is some area of your life you'd like to improve, please consider this exercise. Start with just one person. Remember, nobody is asking you to trust everyone. That would be foolish. Many people are untrustworthy, but, contrary to your belief, not *everyone* is. Your job is to discern who is/are the exception to the rule.

Keep these ideas in mind as you consider who truly belongs where as you complete your circles. Your first task is to think about all the people in your life and where they go in your circles. Then consider the questions that follow to get you started making healthy changes to your relationships. Work with your therapist or other helping professional if you need ongoing guidance or accountability.

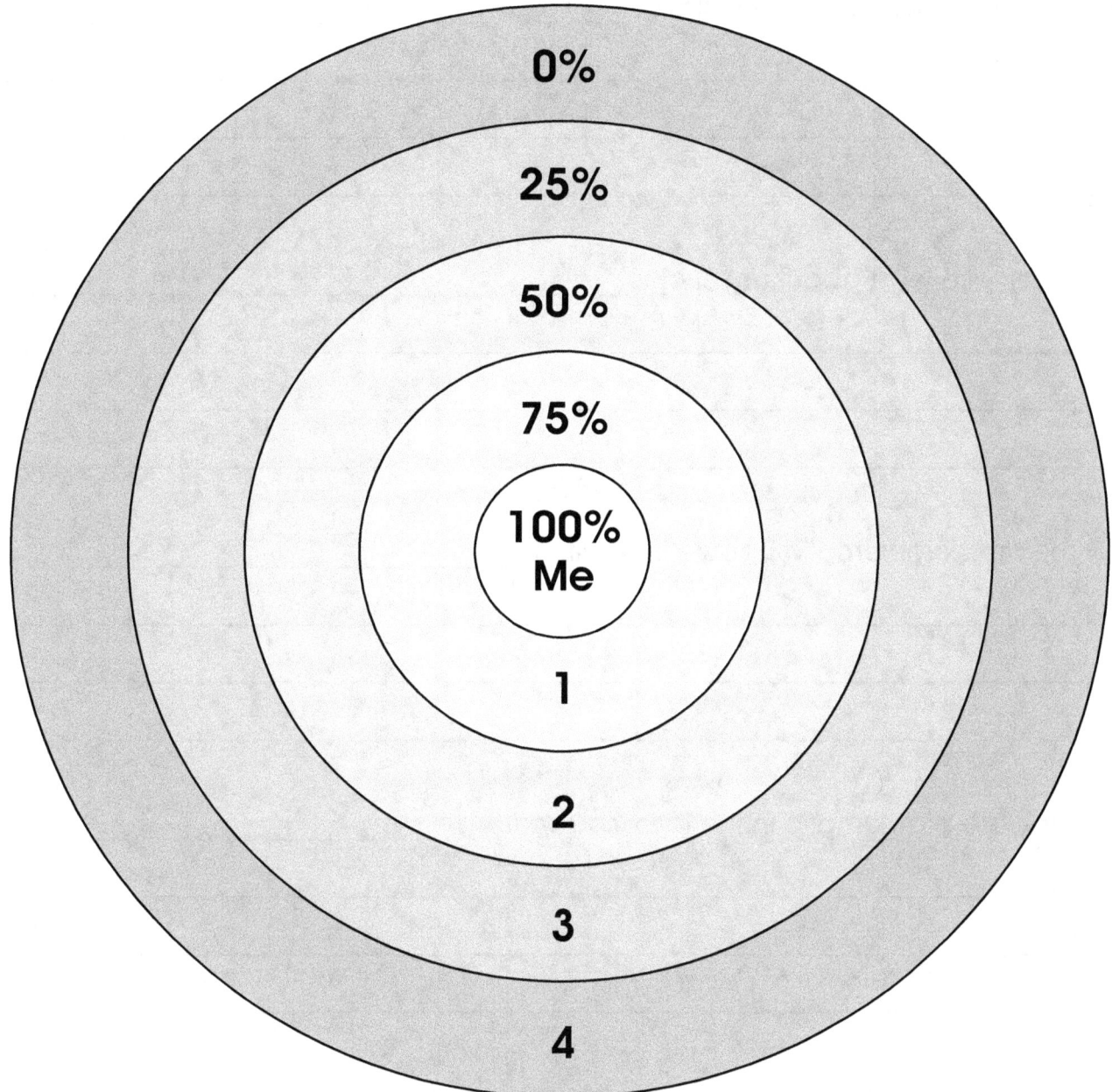

Intimacy Circles Follow-Up Starter Questions

- General observations about my circles _____
_____
_____
_____

Chapter 8: The Paranoid Personality Disorder

- What I like most about my circles _____
  _____
  _____
  _____

- What I like least about my circles _____
  _____
  _____
  _____

- The most problematic people in my life _____
  _____
  _____
  _____

- They are problematic in the following ways _____
  _____
  _____
  _____

- People in my life whose opinions I actually care about and on a scale of 0-10 how much I care what they think _____
  _____
  _____
  _____

- People in my life whose opinions I don't care about _____
  _____
  _____

- People in my life whom I have hurt/violated/taken advantage of _____
  _____
  _____
  _____

- People in my life who have moved themselves out in my circles due to my behavior
  _____
  _____
  _____

- I could improve my circles if I were willing to keep the following rules (which I have not previously been willing to keep) _____
  _____
  _____
  _____

- One step I will take TODAY to improve my relationship circles _____
  _____
  _____
  _____

Tool #6: Identify and Restructure Automatic Thoughts

A staple component of treatment for any psychological condition is recognizing the thought processes that are driving the problem behaviors and maintaining the symptoms. In colloquial language, you may hear this referred to as "self-talk." To speak in the terms of the Mark Twain quote in the introduction ("If all you have is a hammer, everything looks like a nail"): This is the "hammer." While treatment of personality disorders requires more tools than just a hammer, the hammer is still a useful tool to have in your toolbox.

Some people develop an awareness of their thoughts and get better at noticing them, but do nothing to change them. For example, if we recognize that we are overweight, but do nothing to change our diets or exercise levels, we will stay overweight. In the same way, if we recognize thoughts that are driving problem behavior but do nothing to change them, our symptoms are likely to remain.

So, one cognitive tool you can use is what is called challenging distorted thoughts when you recognize them. Refer to the beginning of this chapter for some distorted thoughts common in paranoid personality disorder. *"Challenging,"* in this case, basically means "arguing" with the specific content of the thoughts. There are a number of techniques that can be used for doing this, including looking at evidence, seeking input from others, researching the facts, considering past or possible future results, or good old-fashioned logic, just to name a few.

The following tool asks you to identify specific paranoid thoughts that enter your mind, challenge them in some way, and if you want to, rate your challenge on a scale of 0-10, indicating how meaningful the challenge is. Take a look at the example, and then do one on your own. This may be a tool that you will benefit from using on an ongoing basis.

Example: Thought Log

Suspicious Thought	Rational Responses
Since that policeman made eye contact with me in the bakery, he probably knows I was speeding on the way here and is here to arrest me	He might have not really been looking at me (1) Maybe he just was making eye contact to be polite (0) Most people make eye contact with people they come in contact with; – I it might have meant nothing (4) He probably doesn't even know I was speeding on the way here (1) Speeding is not a violation to arrest someone over—I won't go to jail (5)

Analysis: This client is a highly suspicious young man. You might note here he is *less* likely to endorse ideas related to the notion that the policeman was *not* there for him specifically. His highest believability rating was given to a challenge that asked him to examine the severity of the consequences. It is common with paranoid individuals to give higher believably ratings to the "even if it did happen" or the "what does that have to mean?" challenges than the "it probably won't happen" challenges.

My Paranoid Thought Log

Suspicious Thoughts	Rational Responses

Tool #7: Historical Experiences Worksheet

As with most, if not all personality disorders, there are multiple pathways to PPD. Very few people with PPD present themselves in clinical and coaching settings, for obvious reasons. Thus, similar to histrionic and dependent PDs, there is no large scale research here. However a few commonalities in backgrounds of experience have been observed. Peruse the following historical experiences worksheet and put an "X" beside factors that were a part of your experiences from a young age.

- ☐ History of being humiliated or embarrassed in some significant way
- ☐ History of multiple hurts as child
- ☐ Parents were highly punitive
- ☐ Raised in a family where anger was outwardly displayed with frequency
- ☐ Families were not open and intimacy was never modeled

- Describe how the experiences checked above apply specifically to you and the impact you believe they continue to have in your life today

_____
_____
_____
_____
_____
_____
_____
_____
_____
_____

Tool #8: Belief Identification

As has been discussed, all behaviors are a product of beliefs. Beliefs drive behavior. Due to the compelling nature of beliefs in individuals with PDs, these deeper-level beliefs often have to be modified to help create lasting change. As noted at the beginning of this chapter, common beliefs in people with PPD include mistrust, vulnerability, and punitiveness, among others. Review their definitions if you don't have them fresh in your mind. Get with your therapist. Include friends and family who are willing to give you feedback. Identify one or two beliefs that you believe drive your target behaviors to work on in treatment. Write them inside Judy Beck's "Pac-Man" visual aid (which was explained in the introduction).

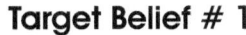 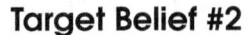

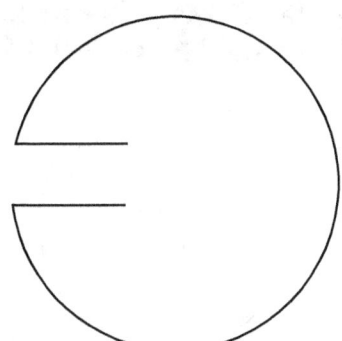 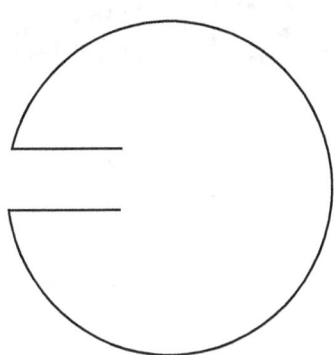

Beliefs always come in pairs. For every maladaptive (or unhealthy) belief we possess, we also possess an alternate, adaptive (or healthy) belief. For instance, even though an individual may have the belief, "Others are untrustworthy," they also have the belief, however faint, "Maybe others can be trusted."

I have given you the "pushing buttons" language, the "Pac-Man" visual, and the "filters" imagery. Here is another representation which I hope helps illustrate the point: We could think of beliefs as lenses. For people who wear glasses, this visual probably comes fairly intuitively. Healthier individuals are able to engage in more balanced information processing. Figuratively speaking they are able to see out of both the left and the right "lenses" equally. This is the goal of belief modification work: balanced information processing. In other words, to be able to see both sides objectively and to be able to recognize when they fail or make mistakes, so they can learn from them; and also to be able to acknowledge when they succeed and be able to take a compliment. Although nobody is perfect and everyone has their biases, healthier people's lenses are closer to the 50/50 range (50% failure/50% success). Before treatment, people with PDs, due to their more compelling beliefs, often start with numbers such as 99%/1%. ***Intentional and sustained effort*** is required to create a healthier belief balance.

So, now that you have identified your unhealthy beliefs driving your target behaviors, identify in your own words what you would call the opposite, healthy belief. Write it in the opposite belief structure that the "triangle" could fit into.

After you have identified your one or two healthy and unhealthy beliefs, ask yourself: "What percentage of the time do I believe the unhealthy belief? What percentage of the time do I believe the healthy belief?" Write your numbers in the line next to each belief (they should total 100%). Then you are ready to move on to Tool #9!

See the example first, and then do one on your own!

Example: Belief Identification

Target Belief #1	Healthy Belief #1
"Others are untrustworthy" 99% Strength	"Some can be trusted" 1% Strength
Target Belief #2	**Healthy Belief #2**
Strength	Strength

My Beliefs

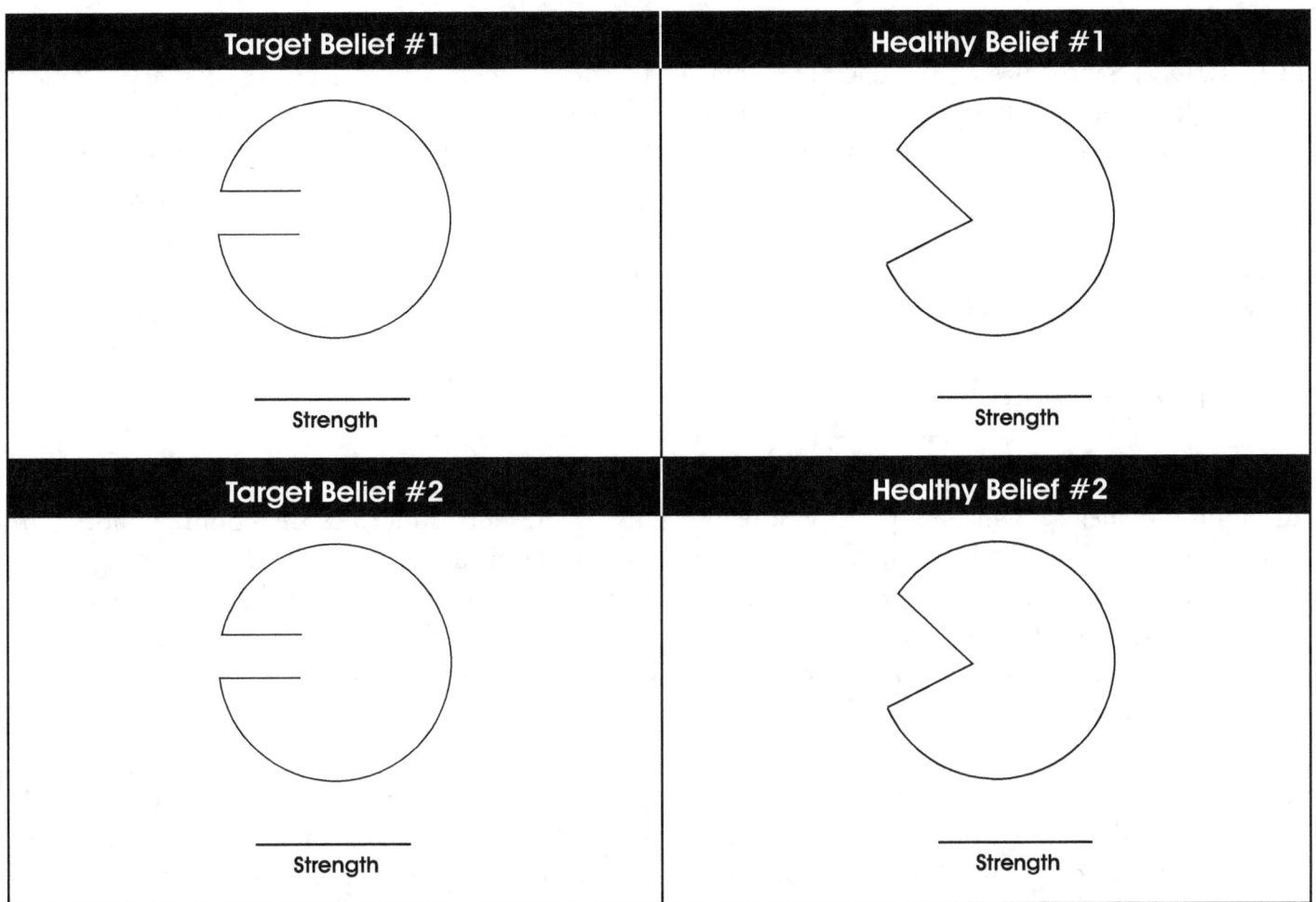

Tool #9: Evidence Logs

Here is where the hard work begins! This is a tool you will use throughout your treatment, regardless of what other tools you may be using and at what stage of treatment you may be at. This is the tough, tough work of gradually working to develop your healthy belief. How do we change beliefs, anyway? It's a difficult process, no doubt. What we need to do is to *reexamine historical evidence, get better at noticing current evidence* **and** *intentionality initiate ongoing experiences around which to create new evidence.*

Think of any belief that you have changed over time in any area of your life. Maybe you used to not believe in God and now you do. Perhaps you used to not believe in global warming and now you do. Maybe you used to believe in life on other planets and now you don't. For example, I have a client who is a marine biology major in college – his chief interest is in Megalodon sharks, which he was initially convinced were not extinct. After a lot of scientific research, he now no longer believes that. Did you used to hold more conservative political beliefs, and your beliefs are now more progressive? You get the gist. You can use a belief that you have changed in *any* area of life to illustrate this process. How do

beliefs change? By examining the evidence created by experience and the meaning that we assign to it.

Take a belief many people once held. (WARNING! UPCOMING CONTENT NOT APPROPRIATE FOR KIDS!) Santa Claus is not real. If you believed in his existence when you were six years old, what was the "evidence" that supported your belief? He brought presents. They said "from Santa" on the wrapping. He drank the milk that was set out for him. He knew what presents were desired from the letters that was sent to him at the North Pole. The local weather even tracks him on the Doppler radar!

Over time, most people reexamine the pieces of evidence and assign new meaning to them. By doing so, they change their belief.

But they have to *experience* new evidence.

Some children recognize Papa beneath the Santa suit and false white beard. Some children stay up all night and sneak downstairs to catch a parent putting presents under the tree. Some children are observant enough to notice that "Santa" has Mommy's identical hand writing or wrapping paper. The child who *does not go out of their way to look for these things* holds onto the old, false belief much longer because they are not looking for evidence to the contrary. In fact, when I myself was becoming suspicious but desperately wanted to believe that he was real as a child, I began actively searching out confirmation of his existence.

In the same way, for any of us to change our beliefs, we must be *willing* to examine evidence fairly. We are naturally (consciously or unconsciously) looking for evidence to support our existing belief. But we must be equally willing to consider evidence to the contrary as well. This is what the evidence logs do: they provide a tool to facilitate *purposefully looking for evidence* to support the new belief you are attempting to construct. If your current unhealthy belief is that you are a failure, then you are purposefully looking for evidence that you can succeed. For some cognitive behavioral therapy (CBT) exercises, we will ask people to log evidence on *both* sides. But because people with PDs have such deeply engrained beliefs, their natural tendency will be to see only evidence that supports the current belief. So, for the purpose of this exercise, it is important to use the right column only to log evidence that supports the belief. The left column will remain blank.

As you record the evidence, think about how it felt to have that experience. As you do, ask yourself: *In this moment* how much do I believe _____ and how much do I believe _____?
                                          (unhealthy belief)   (healthy belief)

Remember, you will inherently *not notice* evidence that will be helpful because your filter is directing you away from it, so be vigilant. Also, when you log evidence for a healthy belief, you will get that little voice in your head that says, "but… it doesn't count because of this or that." Go ahead and record the evidence anyway even if you have trouble believing it at the time.

Log the believability rating as you record each piece of evidence. Note that these numbers will go up

and down, because beliefs fluctuate. But over time, watch your unhealthy numbers generally trend down and your healthy numbers trend up. The more they change, the more balanced your lenses will be come and you will get your "buttons pushed" less frequently!

Look at the example below. Then begin completing your own evidence log, working on one belief at a time. When you have more than one icebergs to conquer, the more effort you put into chiseling one at a time, the more progress you will make.

Example: Evidence Log

Unhealthy Belief: 99%   **Healthy Belief: 1%**

Date	"Others are untrustworthy"	% Belief	"Some can be trusted"	% Belief
1/3		98%	Jacob kept his promise	2%
1/10		95%	Mom picked me up when she said she would	5%
1/16		97%	Police didn't come to my house like I thought they would	3%
1/18		95%	I went for a walk in the park and nothing happened	5%
1/20		78%	I did not get kicked out of treatment like I thought I was going to	22%

Conclusions: I guess there have been a few times that I've been wrong when I was certain I was right, I was okay in all instances

My Evidence Log

Unhealthy Belief: _____   **Healthy Belief:** _____

Date		% Belief		% Belief

Conclusions _____

_____

Tool #10: Distinguishing Dangerous Situations

As stated above, people with PPD believe the world is a scary place and every situation inherently is dangerous. To be fair, many situations in our world today *are* dangerous. Some people actually err on the other end of the spectrum by believing that *no* situations are dangerous. People who believe the best in others often experience the very thing suspicious people fear and guard against the most: getting hurt. One does not have to have a psychiatric disorder to give someone the benefit of the doubt when the doubt has been long gone for years. So your suspiciousness has merit (you already believe that strongly, of course—you don't need me to tell you that). However, as you hopefully discovered in your "pros and cons" exercise, there are definitely disadvantages to being on your end of the spectrum.

So, while it is okay to believe that a lot of the world is dangerous, the challenge is to discern what truly makes a situation dangerous and to be able to identify exceptions. Use the tool below to identify a situation (not a specific person—the next tool will address this) that you perceived as dangerous. It will then ask you to break down what you viewed as dangerous about it and see if you are able to identify themes in your thinking, as well as challenge you to think differently in the future.

"Dangerous Situations" Tool

Describe a past dangerous situation
Elements that made it dangerous
Recurring themes in situations I view as dangerous
What I look for to assess the safety of a situation

Conclusions _____
_____
_____

Tool #11: Qualities of Trust

Okay, now that you have looked at non-personal dangerous situations that occur in your world, this next tool will ask you to do essentially the same thing, except with regard to qualities in people. Likely the left column will come easy to you, but be specific. When you get to the right column, really think hard about specific attributes. Think about someone in your life that you trust now or have trusted in the past. And remember, trust is not an all-or-nothing thing either; perhaps on a scale of 0-10 you trust most people a 0, but you have (or have had) a person in your life that you trusted at "4 or a 5." Think about them and the qualities they have (or had). See how many you can come up with for the right-hand column.

Qualities of Untrustworthy People	Qualities of Trustworthy People

Tool #12: Trust Me!

Here's where the rubber meets the road. Pick a person or two in your life whom you identified in Tool #5 as belonging somewhere in your "circles" that indicates at least some (even if minimal) level of trust. Then take some of the qualities you identified in the previous tool. Watch that person closely (you should be good at that ☺); but instead of watching for what your filters will naturally incline you to, try to be intentional about observing them act in ways that demonstrate one of the qualities you trust. As you observe them being trustworthy, notice how it feels. Notice whether your physiology is different. Notice whether your emotions are different. And, *in that moment*, record on a scale of 0-10 how much you trust that particular person. Logging these ratings over time can build up some trust. And trusting one or two people, even a little bit, can go a long way. You can still distrust most people in life but significantly improve your general well-being.

Person	Trustworthy Behavior Observed	Trust Level in this Moment (0-10)

Tool #13: Anger Management

Anger is one of the dominant emotions dealt with by those suffering from PPD. Many are able to keep their anger to themselves, but explosive outbursts in response to perceived threats can be quite intense. Therefore, some basic anger management (not the Jack Nicholson/Adam Sandler kind) can be beneficial.

There is nothing new or original about this tool. In fact, people have probably been using the time-out technique for centuries. It is most commonly associated with modifying children's behavior, but it may be one of the most important strategies for managing anger for adults as well. The inability to use this technique in heated moments has resulted in hurt feelings, wounded relationships, terminations of employment, destruction of property, and prison sentences.

Many people can recognize how this may be helpful in times when they are not "in the moment," but then prove themselves incapable of using it in times when they really need to. Using this tool requires some degree of mastery of previous tools, including self-monitoring. If we do not realize how angry we are getting or what behaviors our dysfunctional thoughts are tempting us to do, we often don't realize until it's too late. For this reason, awareness of one's anger style is important. For instance, if you are a person whose anger builds slowly over time, you probably can afford to postpone taking a time-out longer than others. Conversely, if you are an impulsive person who can go from zero to sixty in a matter of seconds, so to speak, it is probably more important for you to take a time-out, even as early as when you recognize that your anger is a 1 or a 2.

- The person or situation that is most likely to trigger my anger to the point of having to take a time-out _____

_____

_____

- Steps I could take to prevent the situation from even presenting itself, while still doing things that are important to me _____

_____

_____

Tips for Taking a Time-Out

- **Do** remove yourself from the upsetting situation before you act in a way that could create unwanted consequences.

- **Do** stay away long enough to "cool down." In some cases, this may mean an hour. Other circumstances may require staying away for a day or more.

- **Don't** use alcohol or drugs while in your time-out.

- **Do** use distraction initially. Force yourself to think about something else to help decrease your level of physical arousal so that you can think more clearly. It is important not to tell yourself "Don't think about this," as that makes it likely you will continue to dwell on it. Rather, identify other things with which to consume your thoughts. Examples could include planning a vacation, surfing the internet, counting to 100, or immersing yourself in a movie, football game, or other visual activity that requires your attention.

- If you aren't able to concentrate, **do** something physical: go for a walk, run, or bike ride, do some gardening—anything physical can be helpful.

- Once you calm down, **do** try to think rationally about how to resolve the situation.

- If necessary, **do** consult a friend or person you trust.

- **Do** get validated. Find someone who can validate your feelings, understand where you are coming from, and constructively encourage you how to respond.

- **Don't** find "yes men" (or "yes women") who will fuel your "shoulds." These people seem validating initially but only serve to add fuel to the fire and make us more angry at the person we are already angry at—which is not helpful in the long run, especially if we want or need to maintain an ongoing relationship with that person.

- **Don't** use the time-out as an excuse to completely avoid situations that need to be dealt with. The purpose of the time-out is to temporarily remove yourself so you can go back and deal with the situation, not to permanently avoid it. Many people try to avoid dealing with such situations, but this keeps conflict unresolved and allows anger to continue to simmer.

- If I would have to take a time-out, the following ideas above could be helpful for me _____

- My Time-out Plan

    1. _____
    2. _____
    3. _____
    4. _____
    5. _____

Tool #14: Paranoid Schema Mode Tool

Practitioners of schema therapy have noted that people with PDs have some specific themes in their "states of being" that can include moods and behaviors that are distinct from the run-of-the-mill mood swings that all people have. They have called these state-like experiences schema *modes*. These can be triggered on a moment's notice, and specific modes have distinct characteristics. Certain constellations of beliefs and modes are associated with different PDs. Four modes commonly associated with PPD are:

1. **Paranoid Over-Controller Mode** – In this state, the person attempts to protect oneself from a perceived or real threat by focusing all attention on it and exercising extreme control over it. Some go out of their way in an attempt to locate unseen threats.

2. **Angry Protector Mode** - In this state, people experience intense anger, but it is controlled. They are able to use it as a "wall" to protect themselves. This is often done in isolation by paranoid individuals.

3. **Enraged Child Mode** – Here the anger is no longer hidden behind a "wall." The person loses control when triggered and attacks others or throws the adult version of a child's temper tantrum.

4. **Bully Mode** – This state is similar to the previous, but here, rather than being triggered and reacting to feeling "snuck up on," actions are pre-meditated. The person purposely goes out of their way to retaliate using threats, domineering, bullying language, or physical aggression.

If you have PPD, likely most, if not all, of these "parts" exist somewhere within you. Use the tool to describe specific behavior you have engaged in that you recognize as indicative of the above modes.

- Paranoid Over-Controller Mode _____
_____
_____
_____
_____

- Angry Protector Mode _____
_____
_____
_____
_____

- Enraged Child Mode _____
_____
_____
_____
_____

- Bully Mode _____
_____
_____
_____
_____

- The mode I most relate with _____

- One step I will take to work on these behaviors _____

Tool #15: Forgiveness

Many people hear the term "forgiveness" and are immediately turned off. However, think about it this way: Reluctance to forgive is essentially the same thing as resentment. One is a "spiritual" word and one is more of an "emotional" one (and thus is more acceptable to non-religious or non-spiritual people, some of which are easily offended), but they mean basically the same thing: *anger held onto*. Where I come from, that's also called a grudge. Excessive unforgiving/grudge-holding is actually within DSM criteria for PPD. So if you are turned off by this topic and think it is not for you, you are wrong. This is specifically for you!

Thousands of books have been written on the topic of forgiveness. Comprehensively covering this subject is far outside the scope of this tool. However, examining the role that forgiveness can play in grudge-holding and unresolved anger can be a powerful tool of recovery.

Most major world religions emphasize the benefits of forgiveness Why? Probably because it's good for us! But if it is so obviously good for us, why do so many people resist it? There are many distorted thoughts associated with unwillingness to initiate the practice of forgiveness. Identifying and rationally responding to some of these common abjections is the goal of this tool. Observe the example, then identify some of the internal stumbling blocks that are hindering you from beginning a healthy process that could provide you much relief. Once you break through some of the myths related to forgiveness, you can initiate your own process in your own way.

Example: Forgiveness Thought Log

Distorted Unforgiveness	Rational Response
I will not give him the satisfaction of my forgiveness	Forgiveness is not for them—it is for me. The old adage says, "Unforgiveness is like swallowing a drop of poison every day waiting for the other person to die." I will not continue to give him control over my life now that I have a choice.
Forgiveness is like saying what she did to me is okay	Forgiveness is not saying that at all. Forgiveness is saying what they did is still as unacceptable as it was on the day they did it to me, but I am choosing not to hold it against them any longer—for my own sake.
Forgive and forget—and since I don't think I can forget, then I must not be able to forgive	There are some things in life I will never forget. Actually, if I forget, I may not learn from past situations. Just because I will never forget has nothing to do with my ability to forgive.
If I forgive him, that means I have to trust him again, and there's no way that's happening	Forgiveness is about the past. Trust is about the future. I can forgive him but never trust him again. Forgiveness is always healthy for me, regardless of his behavior, but trust is earned. I can forgive and still set whatever boundaries I want for him.
I'm just not ready to forgive yet—I'll forgive when I feel like it	Anger comes from "shoulds." Forgiving means working to give up my "shoulds." So, until I start working on it, I'll never get around to feeling like it. Forgiveness is first granted, then felt.
I'll forgive her when she apologizes to me	It may be easier if she apologizes, but what if she never does? If I tell myself I will not take steps to better myself until she does—and perhaps she never will—then I'm continuing to give her the power to keep me miserable. I will no longer give her that.
Time heals all wounds. I don't have to do anything—it will just get better with time	Time can help me think about a situation more objectively, but the reality is I can hold a grudge as long as I want to. If time were all it took, no one would go to their grave angry. If I don't want to be one of those people, I have to actually initiate and participate in the forgiveness process. It takes work, but it will be worth it.

Now, identify and rationally respond to your own distorted thoughts which are preventing you from beginning your process of forgiveness.

My Forgiveness Thought Log

Distorted Unforgiveness	Rational Response

Once you have dealt with the thoughts that may have kept you from beginning the process of forgiveness, you are ready to start. People practice forgiveness in many ways. Some steps you may want to consider to get you started are as follows (but are not limited to these):

Example: Forgiveness Steps:

1. Journal
2. Pray
3. Meditate
4. Talk to my therapist
5. Talk to my priest
6. Challenge my "shoulds" daily
7. Practice acceptance
8. Try to empathize
9. Go to church
10. Get reinvolved with my support group and sponsor

My Forgiveness Steps

1. _____
2. _____
3. _____
4. _____
5. _____
6. _____
7. _____
8. _____
9. _____
10. _____

CHAPTER 9: THE BORDERLINE PERSONALITY DISORDER

The Borderline Personality Disorder

Hidden agenda: To not be left

Prevalence rates: Approximately 3% of the general population

Gender distribution: More commonly diagnosed in women than men

Cognitive profile:

- View of self: "I can't be okay alone," "I am defective"

- View of others: "Others will leave me," "Others are wonderful," "Others are untrustworthy" Others will always let me down," "Others are scum"

- View of world: "The world is a cruel and unsafe place"

Common schemas: Abandonment, defectiveness, approval seeking, subjugation, dependent entitlement, insufficient self-control, punitiveness

Common cognitive distortions: Personalization, discounting the positive, rationalization, "should statements" (directed toward self and others), magnification

Overdeveloped traits: Demanding or smothering expectations for others, vengefulness

Underdeveloped traits: Self-control, moderation

Whom they date/marry: Other BPD individuals, antisocials, dependents

Where they work: Nursing, social work

Other Random Nuggets: Most common personality disorder in clinical setting; comprises 20% of psychiatric inpatients

Continuum

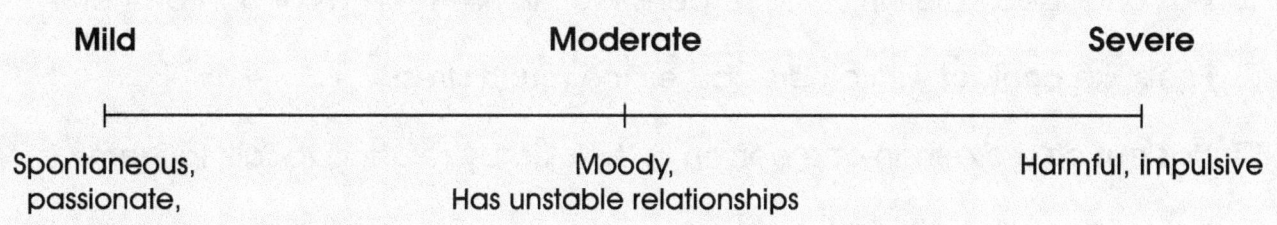

Tool #1: Trait Checklist

Individuals that suffer from the characteristics of borderline personality disorder (BPD) have a number of commonalities. Whether you are a loved one has this full blown condition, or some of the traits of it, survey the following checklist. The more of these you check yes to, the more likely it is this pattern of behavior is causing some problems occupationally, relationally, or socially.

- ❑ Terrified that those closest to them will leave
- ❑ Becomes close to others quickly, but relationships (romantic/family/friends) tend to end abruptly and painfully
- ❑ Ends relationships prematurely so others do not end them first
- ❑ May form positive first impressions of others only to quickly change feelings toward that person to hatred or disinterest
- ❑ Takes on the values, hobbies, or behaviors of those around them rather than holding on to the things that they truly believe and enjoy
- ❑ Feels like there is a "black hole" (i.e., completely empty) inside
- ❑ Feels lonely even when in a relationship or among people who they know love them
- ❑ Experiences multiple intense mood swings in a given day
- ❑ Has trouble being alone
- ❑ Experiences intense emotions related to guilt, self-hatred, self-loathing, or shame

❏ Experiences episodes of rage that are often followed by feelings of guilt and shame

❏ Has engaged in self-injury in response to intense feelings of guilt or shame

❏ Feels like contact with others causes too much stress

❏ Has cut off more than one person in their life by refusing to talk to them

❏ Has engaged in alcohol or drug use, promiscuous sex, binge eating, reckless driving, or shopping sprees in an impulsive manner in order to "numb out," feel better, or create a "rush"

❏ Continually does risky things on the spur of the moment

❏ Has felt as though they did not even exist

❏ Constantly changes ideas about who they are, their career, hobbies, and/or beliefs

❏ Has cut, burned, or otherwise hurt themselves on *purpose but with no intent to die*

❏ Has been accused by others of being paranoid

❏ Has experienced periods of time they can't account for, or has been faced with evidence for doing something which they don't remember doing

Tool #2: Expressions of Concern

All people have what are often called "blind spots": qualities we don't see in ourselves as well as others see in us. Because of the ego-syntonic nature of PDs, this phenomenon is particularly challenging for these people. What this means practically is that things that pose problems for friends and family members are often not are considered problematic by the individual with the condition. Concerns expressed by friends and family may have validity to them, but due to poor insight, the PD individual generally has difficulty seeing how certain behaviors impact themselves or others negatively. However, not all concerns friends and family express have validity. So, one of the tough but vital steps for recovery is sorting through these "complaints" to determine which ones have validity and which do not. One issue that arises with this exercise is that individuals with borderline personality disorder (BPD) tend to overvalue certain persons' opinion and undervalue others'.

Use the following tool to identify *who* has expressed concern, *what* the exact concerns are, and *why* they see them as potentially hurtful. Look at the example, then complete your own and answer the questions that follow.

Example:

Person Expressing Concern	Action Causing Concern	Reason for Concern
1. Cari (friend)	1. Cutting	1. Might accidentally cut too deep and die
2. Mom	2. Alcohol use	2. Alcoholism; health concerns
3. JoAnn (pastor)	3. Promiscuous sex	3. Self-image
4. Crissy (friend)	4. Current boyfriend abusive?	4. Physical/emotional safety
5. Aunt	5. Meth	5. Psychologically damage my kids

Questions:

- Who are three people I trust to "shoot straight" with me, by whom I can run these concerns to get their opinion?

    1. Aunt

    2. Boyfriend

    3. JoAnn

- With which concerns can I at least see where the person is coming from?

    Alcohol use – I barely drink – I am not going to become an alcoholic or have health problems

- Which concerns can I see the most validity in?

    I really don't want to psychologically damage my kids

- I am willing to take the following steps to change one of the concerns
    1. Go to therapy
    2. Not use Meth again
    3. Not return Jeremy's messages (drug dealer)

My Expressions of Concern

Person Expressing Concern	Action Causing Concern	Reason for Concern
1.	1.	1.
2.	2.	2.
3.	3.	3.
4.	4.	4.
5.	5.	5.

Questions:

- Who are three people I trust to "shoot straight" with me, by whom I can run these concerns by to get their opinion?

    1. _____
    2. _____
    3. _____

- With which concerns can I at least see where the person is coming from? _____
_____
_____

- Which concerns can I see the most validity in? _____
_____

- I am willing to take the following steps to change one of the concerns

    1. _____

    2. _____

    3. _____

Tool #3: Pros and Cons

This tool helps you evaluate the potential pros and cons of your destructive, impulsive behaviors. It is called a *four-box pros and cons*. Sometimes it can be beneficial to look at not only the advantages and disadvantages of maintaining certain behaviors but also the advantages and disadvantages of changing them. After listing the pros and cons of each, it can be even more helpful to rate on a scale of 0-10 how important each item is. Consider the example that is provided. Then complete one on your own.

Example: Pros and Cons of Destructive/Impulsive Behavior

Pros of Continuing Destructive/Impulsive Behavior (Example: Cutting)	Pros of Developing Self-Control and Treating Self Well
Calms me down when I get manic (10)	No scars (6) No looks in public (7) Treated better by doctors (9) No more infections (8)
Cons of Continuing Destructive/Impulsive Behavior (Example: Cutting)	**Cons of Developing Self-Control and Treating Self Well**
More scars (6) Could accidentally bleed out (10) More infections (8) More doctors and hospitals (10)	No way to cope with intense emotions if skills don't work (9) Stay in emotional pain (9)

Results:

__10__ Reasons to continue impulsive/destructive behavior

__34__ Reasons to not continue impulsive/destructive behavior

__30__ Reasons to develop self-control and treat self well

__18__ Reasons to not develop self-control and treat self well

My Conclusions: It is clearly worth it to me to not cut

My Commitment:

1. Move my coping card to my cutting spot

2. Commit to wait fifteen minutes before acting and try three other skills off my card during that time, call my therapist at minute fourteen

Analysis: It should first be noted that this female client does not have bipolar disorder and does not experience true manic episodes. This book just uses real illustrations with real client language. "Manic" was just a word she used colloquially for when she experienced intense emotions of any kind. It is also noteworthy that she only had one "pro" for engaging in the behavior—it simply was such a strong one, and she had never explored alternatives at that point, so she saw no other way to cope. In terms of the whole exercise, she clearly saw how cutting was not best for her. Her task is now one of recognizing triggers better, tolerating intense emotions, and using skills to decrease her "mania" with less damaging consequences.

My Pros and Cons of Destructive/Impulsive Behavior

Pros of Continuing Destructive/Impulsive Behavior	Pros of Developing Self-Control and Treating Self Well
Cons of Continuing Destructive/Impulsive Behavior	**Cons of Developing Self-Control and Treating Self Well**

Results:

_____ Reasons to continue impulsive/destructive behavior

_____ Reasons to not continue impulsive/destructive behavior

_____ Reasons to develop self-control and treat self well

_____ Reasons to not develop self-control and treat self

My Conclusions _____

_____

_____

_____

My Commitment(s) _____

_____

_____

Tool #4: Identify Behavioral Targets

BPD manifests differently in different people, and in a wider variety of ways than most PDs. This likely contributes to the frequency with which it is misdiagnosed. Common behaviors include intense environmentally triggered (usually relationally triggered) mood swings, impulsive spending, sex, screaming, substance use, unusually fast or reckless driving. It can include jumping from one relationship to the next, or, conversely, staying in unhealthy relationships for extended periods of time. It can include taking on the hobbies or interests of others. It can include self-injury or suicidal threats or attempts.

Use this tool to identify some of your borderline behaviors that you or others have noticed. Feel free to use any of the above behaviors that fit, or list some of your own.

- Behaviors related to my borderline traits that I or someone else identified which I am willing to target to improve my situation

    1. _____
    2. _____
    3. _____
    4. _____
    5. _____

Tool #5: Intimacy Circles

Intimacy is a scary word for a lot of people. If the sound of it makes you cringe, this exercise is definitely for you—and even if it doesn't, this exercise likely will still benefit you. It will benefit almost everyone in some way. Why? Because almost everyone could benefit from improving at least one interpersonal relationship in their life. Some people's lives could be enriched with more friends. Others need to learn to set boundaries with someone in their life. A lot of people have "trust issues." Yet others would be happier in life if they learned to pick healthier people to date or form friendships with; toxic people have a way of draining people of their energy and joy. A certain percentage of the population would be much less prone to mood swings if they could be okay alone. Some would find more fulfillment in life if they could share more with people in their lives; others would not be hurt as often if they learned to share less with those in their life. A lot of people walk around with their "walls" up. Some have difficulty expressing feelings. Some have been accused of being too "needy." Others have difficulty asking for help.

You may have heard intimacy defined as "Into-Me-See"—the degree to which we let people see into us, and vice versa. A lot of my clients have found this "play on words" to be a helpful way to remember its definition and connotations.

Use the following tool to evaluate the relationships in your life. Use the percentage signs to help you decide which people to put in which circles. No other person goes in the ME circle (though some people choose to put God here). This is for you alone. People who belong in circle #1 are those with whom you would feel comfortable sharing ANY problem in life, no matter how personal (a sexual problem, something related to an abusive situation, a salary issue, etc.). People in circle #2 are those in your life with whom there may be a personal issue or two (like the ones mentioned above) that you would not share, but you would be comfortable sharing ALMOST anything (roughly 75%) about your life. People in circle #3 may get about half of your personal stuff, but the other half you probably would not trust them with. People in circle #4 would be your very casual relationships. Maybe they know whether you are married or where you work or something of that nature, but you don't share very much with them (roughly 25%). And people in circle #5 get nothing. For some people, these are individuals whom they have just met, so they could be candidates to move closer in as they get to know them. Or, these are people who at one point in life were closer in, but they have done something to violate trust, so they have had to be moved out one or more rings.

Interpersonal relationships can be very problematic for persons with BPD. Most people with intense emotions desperately feel that they need relationships. Thus, many with BPD or other relational disorders often attempt to develop relationships very quickly and tend to place trust that fosters intimacy in relationships sooner than is wise, considering how little they really know the other person. Many, then, get hurt in relationships, and eventually get hurt so many times that trusting again is difficult. Therefore, some people with these issues put up "walls" that keep others from getting in. These walls function in the sense that they keep people from getting in to hurt them; however, they keep people from getting in to help them as well. On the other hand, others with BPD never put up walls and continue to seek and cultivate relationships throughout their lives, that remain intense, volatile and painful.

Keep these ideas in mind as you consider who truly belongs where as you complete your circles. Your first task is to think about all the people in your life and where they go in your circles. Then consider the questions that follow to get you started making healthy changes to your relationships. Work with your therapist or other helping professional if you need ongoing guidance or accountability.

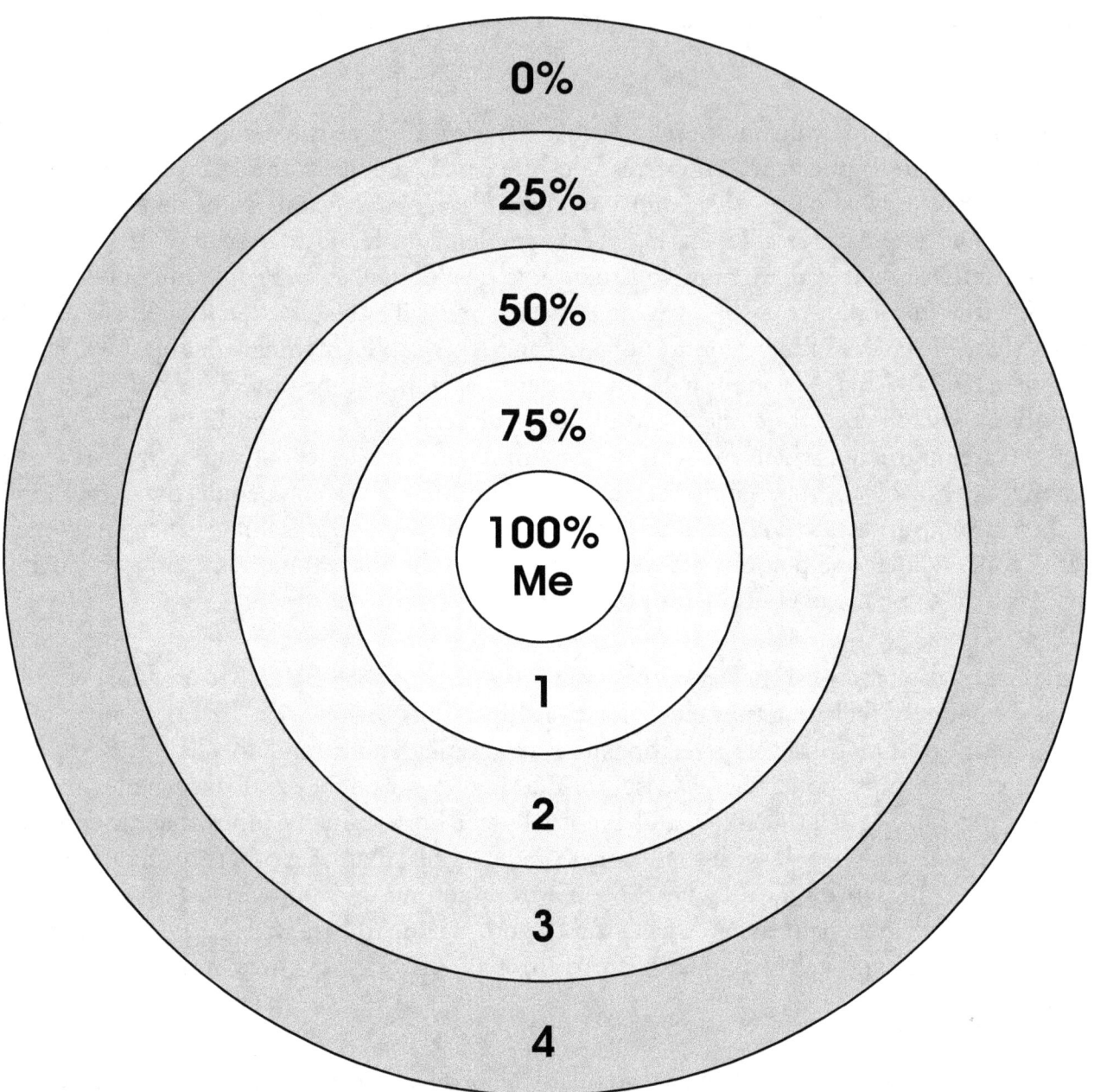

Intimacy Circles Follow-Up Starter Questions

- General observations about my circles _____
_____
_____
_____

- What I like most about my circles _____
  _____
  _____
  _____

- What I like least about my circles _____
  _____
  _____
  _____

- The most problematic people currently in my life _____
  _____
  _____
  _____

- They are problematic in the following ways _____
  _____
  _____
  _____

- People in my life that have hurt me most _____
  _____
  _____
  _____

- People in my life that I have hurt the most _____
  _____
  _____
  _____

- People in my life that I have moved out of my circle that has been for the better
  _____
  _____
  _____

- People in my life that I have moved out of my circle that I have later regretted
  _____
  _____
  _____

- People in my life that have moved themselves out in my circles due to my behavior
  _____
  _____
  _____

- One pattern I see in **my behavior** that have affected my circles _____
  _____
  _____
  _____

- One step I will take TODAY to improve my current relationship circles _____
  _____
  _____
  _____

Tool #6: Identify and Restructure Automatic Thoughts

A staple component of treatment for any psychological condition is recognizing the thought processes that are driving the problem behaviors and maintaining the symptoms. In colloquial language, you may hear this referred to as "self-talk." To speak in the terms of the Mark Twain quote in the introduction

("If all you have is a hammer, everything looks like a nail"): This is the "hammer." While treatment of personality disorders requires more tools than just a hammer, the hammer is still a useful tool to have in your toolbox.

Some people develop an awareness of their thoughts and get better at noticing them, but do nothing to change them. For example, if we recognize that we are overweight, but do nothing to change our diets or exercise levels, we will stay overweight. In the same way, if we recognize thoughts that are driving problem behavior but do nothing to change them, our symptoms are likely to remain.

So, one cognitive tool you can use is what is called challenging distorted thoughts when you recognize them. Refer to the beginning of this chapter for some distorted thoughts common in borderline personality disorder. *"Challenging,"* in this case, basically means "arguing" with the specific content of the thoughts. There are a number of techniques that can be used for doing this, including looking at evidence, seeking input from others, researching the facts, considering past or possible future results, or good old-fashioned logic, just to name a few.

The following tool asks you to identify specific borderline thoughts that enter your mind, challenge them in some way, and if you want to, rate your challenge on a scale of 0-10, indicating how meaningful the challenge is. Take a look at the example, and then do one on your own. This may be a tool that you will benefit from using on an ongoing basis.

Example: Thought Log

Distorted Thought	Rational Responses
Since she said that, she must not care about me	She might not have meant it like it sounded to me
	Is there any other evidence that she cares about me?
	What things has she done in the last month that might mean she does care?
	Maybe she didn't mean it to sound so direct
	Even if she did, sometimes I need people to be direct with me or I don't hear them
	I could ask her to clarify what she means. She is too good a friend to lose over a possible misinterpretation.

My BPD Thought Log

BPD Thoughts	Rational Responses

Tool #7: Historical Experiences Worksheet

The causes of BPD have been researched more than any other personality disorder. Genetic heritability rates are have been estimated to be just over 50%. While we are still learning about this interplay, it is known that people with BPD are born with a biological predisposition to emotional sensitivity in comparison to other people. This predisposition seems to be necessary to "load the gun" so to speak. Some of the factors below are believed to be involved in "pulling the trigger." Peruse the following historical experiences worksheet and put an "X" beside factors that were a part of your experiences from a young age.

- ❏ Death of a parent
- ❏ Loss of another family member
- ❏ Substance use in family
- ❏ Parents punished expressions of emotions
- ❏ Chaotic home with people regularly "in and out"
- ❏ Family failed to validate emotions or experiences
- ❏ Siblings were often compared to each other
- ❏ Value was not affirmed by parents or caregivers
- ❏ Physical/sexual abuse

- Describe how the experiences checked above apply specifically to you and the impact you believe they continue to have in your life today

_____
_____
_____
_____
_____
_____
_____
_____
_____
_____

Tool #8: Belief Identification

As has been discussed, all behaviors are a product of beliefs. Beliefs drive behavior. Due to the compelling nature of beliefs in individuals with PDs, these deeper-level beliefs often have to be modified to help create lasting change. As noted at the beginning of this chapter, common beliefs in people with BPD include abandonment, defectiveness, approval seeking, punitiveness, subjugation, dependent entitlement, and insufficient self-control. Review their definitions if you don't have them fresh in your mind. Get with your therapist. Include friends and family who are willing to give you feedback. Identify one or two beliefs that you believe drive your target behaviors to work on in treatment. Write them inside Judy Beck's "Pac-Man" visual aid (which was explained in the introduction).

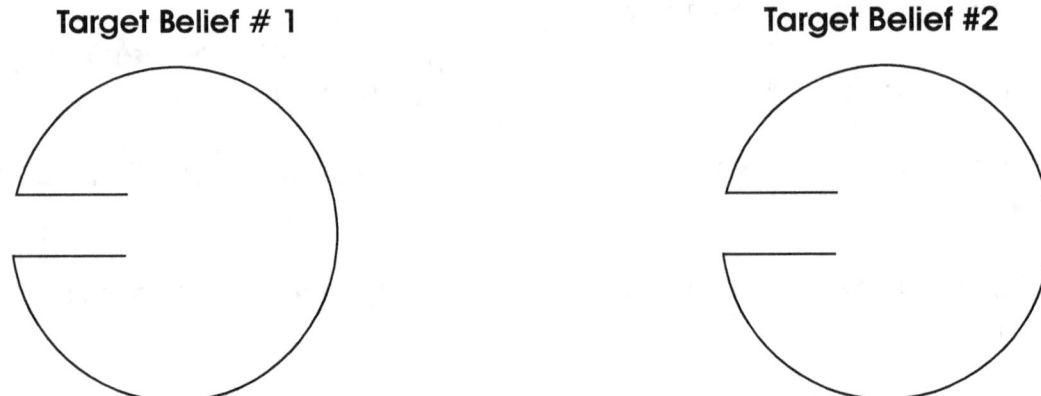

Beliefs always come in pairs. For every maladaptive (or unhealthy) belief we possess, we also possess an alternate, adaptive (or healthy) belief. For instance, even though an individual may have the belief, "I can't be okay alone," they also have the belief, however faint, "I can be okay alone."

I have given you the "pushing buttons" language, the "Pac-Man" visual, and the "filters" imagery. Here is another representation which I hope helps illustrate the point: We could think of beliefs as lenses. For people who wear glasses, this visual probably comes fairly intuitively. Healthier individuals are able to engage in more balanced information processing. Figuratively speaking they are able to see out of both the left and the right "lenses" equally. This is the goal of belief modification work: balanced information processing. In other words, to be able to see both sides objectively and to be able to recognize when they fail or make mistakes, so they can learn from them; and also to be able to acknowledge when they succeed and be able to take a compliment. Although nobody is perfect and everyone has their biases, healthier people's lenses are closer to the 50/50 range (50% failure/50% success). Before treatment, people with PDs, due to their more compelling beliefs, often start with numbers such as 99%/1%. ***Intentional and sustained effort*** is required to create a healthier belief balance.

So, now that you have identified your unhealthy beliefs driving your target behaviors, identify in your own words what you would call the opposite, healthy belief. Write it in the opposite belief structure that the "triangle" could fit into.

After you have identified your one or two healthy and unhealthy beliefs, ask yourself: "What percentage of the time do I believe the unhealthy belief? What percentage of the time do I believe the healthy belief?" Write your numbers in the line next to each belief (they should total 100%). Then you are ready to move on to Tool #9!

See the example first, and then do one on your own!

Example: Belief Identification

Target Belief #1	Healthy Belief #1
"Others will leave me and I can't be okay alone"	"Some will stay and I can be okay"
97% Strength	3% Strength

Target Belief #2	Healthy Belief #2
Strength	Strength

My Beliefs

Target Belief #1	Healthy Belief #1
Strength	Strength
Target Belief #2	**Healthy Belief #2**
Strength	Strength

Tool #9: Evidence Logs

Here is where the hard work begins! This is a tool you will use throughout your treatment, regardless of what other tools you may be using and at what stage of treatment you may be at. This is the tough, tough work of gradually working to develop your healthy belief. How do we change beliefs, anyway? It's a difficult process, no doubt. What we need to do is to *reexamine historical evidence*, *get better at noticing current evidence* **and** *intentionality initiate ongoing experiences around which to create new evidence*.

Think of any belief that you have changed over time in any area of your life. Maybe you used to not believe in God and now you do. Perhaps you used to not believe in global warming and now you do. Maybe you used to believe in life on other planets and now you don't. For example, I have a client who is a marine biology major in college – his chief interest is in Megalodon sharks, which he was initially convinced were not extinct. After a lot of scientific research, he now no longer believes that. Did you used to hold more conservative political beliefs, and your beliefs are now more progressive? You get the gist. You can use a belief that you have changed in *any* area of life to illustrate this process. How do

beliefs change? By examining the evidence created by experience and the meaning that we assign to it.

Take a belief many people once held. (WARNING! UPCOMING CONTENT NOT APPROPRIATE FOR KIDS!) Santa Claus is not real. If you believed in his existence when you were six years old, what was the "evidence" that supported your belief? He brought presents. They said "from Santa" on the wrapping. He drank the milk that was set out for him. He knew what presents were desired from the letters that was sent to him at the North Pole. The local weather even tracks him on the Doppler radar!

Over time, most people reexamine the pieces of evidence and assign new meaning to them. By doing so, they change their belief.

But they have to *experience* new evidence.

Some children recognize Papa beneath the Santa suit and false white beard. Some children stay up all night and sneak downstairs to catch a parent putting presents under the tree. Some children are observant enough to notice that "Santa" has Mommy's identical hand writing or wrapping paper. The child who *does not go out of their way to look for these things* holds onto the old, false belief much longer because they are not looking for evidence to the contrary. In fact, when I myself was becoming suspicious but desperately wanted to believe that he was real as a child, I began actively searching out confirmation of his existence.

In the same way, for any of us to change our beliefs, we must be *willing* to examine evidence fairly. We are naturally (consciously or unconsciously) looking for evidence to support our existing belief. But we must be equally willing to consider evidence to the contrary as well. This is what the evidence logs do: they provide a tool to facilitate *purposefully looking for evidence* to support the new belief you are attempting to construct. If your current unhealthy belief is that you are a failure, then you are purposefully looking for evidence that you can succeed. For some cognitive behavioral therapy (CBT) exercises, we will ask people to log evidence on *both* sides. But because people with PDs have such deeply engrained beliefs, their natural tendency will be to see only evidence that supports the current belief. So, for the purpose of this exercise, it is important to use the right column only to log evidence that supports the belief. The left column will remain blank.

As you record the evidence, think about how it felt to have that experience. As you do, ask yourself: *In this moment* how much do I believe _____ and how much do I believe _____?
               (unhealthy belief)   (healthy belief)

Remember, you will inherently *not notice* evidence that will be helpful because your filter is directing you away from it, so be vigilant. Also, when you log evidence for a healthy belief, you will get that little voice in your head that says, "but… it doesn't count because of this or that." Go ahead and record the evidence anyway even if you have trouble believing it at the time.

Log the believability rating as you record each piece of evidence. Note that these numbers will go up

and down, because beliefs fluctuate. But over time, watch your unhealthy numbers generally trend down and your healthy numbers trend up. The more they change, the more balanced your lenses will become and you will get your "buttons pushed" less frequently!

Look at the example below. Then begin completing your own evidence log, working on one belief at a time. When you have more than one icebergs to conquer, the more effort you put into chiseling one at a time, the more progress you will make.

Example: Evidence Log

Date	Unhealthy Belief: 97% "Others will leave me and I can't be okay alone"	% Belief	Healthy Belief: 3% "Some will stay and I can be okay alone"	% Belief
11/21		97%	Had a fight with my husband and he didn't leave	3%
11/22		85%	My husband worked eight hours and I only texted him twice	15%
11/23		75%	I called my husband a bad name and he stayed	25%
12/1		80%	My husband didn't return my text and I didn't flip out	20%
12/2		70%	My husband glanced at another woman at dinner but I didn't feel hurt as deeply and I didn't flip out like usual	30%

Conclusions: At least one person has given me some evidence they will stand by my side and I am getting a little less needy when they aren't around

My Evidence Log

Date	Unhealthy Belief:	% Belief	Healthy Belief:	% Belief

Conclusions _____

_____

Chapter 9: The Borderline Personality Disorder

Tool #10: Safety Planning

Reasons for Living

First things first. Not all people with BPD have suicidal ideation or commit acts of self-injury. In fact, research suggests perhaps as high as 25% of people with BPD do not. Having said that, the majority do struggle with it. So here we will start in terms of acuity. Dialectical Behavior Therapy (DBT) protocol recommends addressing patient issues in the order of:

1. Life interfering behaviors

2. Therapy interfering behaviors, and

3. Quality of life interfering behaviors

In 1983, Marsha Linehan wrote an article entitled, "Reasons for Living When One is Considering Committing Suicide." When people become truly suicidal, it is not always that they desire to be dead, but rather that they have lost their will to live. A sad fact is that a significant percentage of people with BPD who don't mean to actually die by suicide do as self-destructive behavior. That is, they just feel so bad in any given moment that they will do almost anything to alleviate the pain, and sometimes the coping skill they resort to results in death. Having reasons for living is important for all human beings, but especially so for those who struggle with recurring suicidal thoughts. Since Linehan's article, a number of "reasons for living" inventories have been developed and are available in the public domain. The following is a modified version. Use this tool to identify reasons that it is important for you to continue to live. It is often helpful to have these easily accessible when thoughts of suicide or self-injury recur.

- ❑ I believe that I have a responsibility to my family
- ❑ I believe only God has the right to take a life
- ❑ I am afraid of death
- ❑ I do not believe things are bad enough that I would rather be dead
- ❑ It is against my religious beliefs to kill myself
- ❑ I believe I still have something to offer the world
- ❑ I want to see my children grow up and be there to support them

- ❏ I still have things I want to accomplish in life
- ❏ I am afraid of the unknown
- ❏ There is no evidence that, if I die, I will be in a better place
- ❏ No matter how badly I feel now, I know it will not last
- ❏ I believe life is too sacred to end it
- ❏ I want to experience joy again
- ❏ I am afraid it will not work and I'll become a vegetable
- ❏ I am afraid of going to hell
- ❏ I believe committing suicide would damage my children psychologically
- ❏ I am afraid of the pain
- ❏ I would not want my family to feel guilty afterwards
- ❏ I do not want people to think I was selfish
- ❏ I still have a desire to live

Use the following tool to identify your reasons for living. They can be directly from this list, related to this list, or completely different.

My Reasons for Living

1. _____
2. _____
3. _____
4. _____
5. _____

Safeguard the Environment

Safeguarding the environment is a tool designed for you to separate yourself from the means of acting on your harmful urges. For instance, if your urge is to cut yourself, safeguarding may involve removing any sharp items from the house. If your urge is to overdose on medication, safeguarding may involve allowing a loved one to lock up your medications and dispense it to you when appropriate. If your urge involves use of alcohol, safeguarding may involve removing all alcohol from the house. If your urge involves spending money impulsively that you don't have, safeguarding may involve giving your credit card to your spouse until your urge subsides.

I have a client in my program who struggles with urges to self-injure. Although she has gradually been willing to get rid of the "kit" she has used in the past to harm herself, she refuses to get rid of her one final blade. Her safeguarding at this point involves putting her blade in a glass of ice and freezing it. She still has it, but if she chooses to act on her urge to self-harm, she will have to wait until it thaws. Safeguarding does not guarantee you will not act destructively; it merely delays action, giving you time to think more rationally and change your mind.

Safety Planning

Once you have identified your reasons for living and have safeguarded your environment, it is important to commit to a personal safety plan. Anyone in treatment for BPD should always have a safety plan. It is important to know your plan, have hard copies of your plan, and have at least one other person who knows your plan and can assist you in implementing it in case your that destructive urges recur. A safety plan is not a simple yes or no answer to the statement, "I promise I will be safe." It is much more specific and proactive. It requires that you identify several particular things you promise to do if you have a dangerous urge come over you, rather than acting on that urge. Use the following tool to develop your personal safety plan.

Safety Plan

I, _____, contract for my safety. This means I promise not to act on my thoughts of attempting to hurt myself in any way. Before acting on my urges to harm or kill myself, I agree to:

1. _____

2. _____

3. _____

4. _____

5. _____

Tool #11: Self-Monitoring

Self-monitoring is an important tool to use in managing mental health symptoms in general, but particularly for people with BPD. First, before we can work to change unhelpful traits into helpful ones, we have to recognize when they are occurring. Second, we have to be able to tell whether we are getting better or not. And if we don't know what we are looking for, we don't know how to measure success.

Third, the tool of self-monitoring will help you learn to observe your own feelings and behavior more accurately. Observing and recording feelings and behavior helps immediately, as you can become more aware of when certain emotions are present and what impact each has on your actions. For instance, if we don't even realize a thought is irrational, we would see no need to challenge it.

Perhaps the easiest way to get started is with behaviors which you have no real desire to change. Some people start with going to the bathroom, brushing their teeth, coughing, or eating. Start by observing *frequency* and *duration*; that is, how *often* you do the behavior, and once you do it, how long the behavior continues.

After getting better at noticing everyday behaviors, you can use this emerging skill to monitor your BPD characteristics.

Answer the following questions:

- What are some traits of your BPD that you would like to change? _____
  _____
  _____

- What characteristic would be helpful for you to monitor in order to gauge your progress over time? _____
  _____
  _____

It is important to identify baseline points for some of these markers so that you can track your progress over time. Use the tool below to record some starting points for some of your current traits.

Example: Baseline Points

BPD Trait	How Often It Manifests
Cutting	3x/week
Episode of Rage	4x/week
Feeling intense emotion but shutting down	3-4 x/day
Avoiding healthy people/opportunities	Twice this week

My BPD Trait

BPD Trait	How Often It Manifests

Self-monitoring does not come easily, and most people believe they are better at it than they really are. But the more you practice, the more self-aware you become. The more self-aware you become, the better insight you have into behaviors that you might want to change that could have a profound positive impact on your recovery. It is important to do this on a regular and ongoing basis to get the most from it.

Tool #12: Monitoring Progress

As mentioned above, progress can only be monitored only once you know specifically which behaviors you are looking to decrease. In my more goal-oriented cognitive coaching programs for people with BPD, I am also constantly asking them what behaviors they would like to increase. Some of my clients are tired of hearing my voice utter the words, "arrows up, arrows down." My point is this: Now that you know what behaviors you are watching, you can identify which behaviors you want to see go up, and which ones you want to see go down.

This is important for several reasons, but perhaps the most important two are 1) subjective experience is not a reliable indicator of a person's growth over time, and 2) people with BPD (and likely members of their support system) have been "programmed" to look for negatives.

To briefly address the first point: Since a typical course of treatment for BPD is between one and four years, it is common that clients will say something like "I am checking in today at a "7" and I noticed in my journal that I rated my mood a "7" a year ago at this time." By that logic, it is easy to conclude that one is not getting any better. But the thing to consider is that a "7" today is often not anywhere near what a "7" was a year ago. So, having a little something more objective to look at can be important. This is one of the reason, it is important to purposefully pay attention to behavioral and situational "evidence." People typically get better at noticing and recording this over the course of treatment.

Regarding the second point: I had a client's father call me relatively recently and make the statement on my voicemail: "Stacy cut herself again last night—she has been seeing you for four months and she is still cutting! She isn't any better!" The truth was that she did cut herself, and fairly badly, the previous night. That made me sad, and the circumstances around it certainly needed to be examined closely at her next appointment. However, the statement that "she isn't any better!" was not accurate. When I met Stacy four months previously, she had been cutting herself daily for the past eight years. In four months of treatment, we had decreased this behavior to approximately once every two weeks.

In addition to decreasing the target behavior ("arrows down") we had increased some positive behaviors that contributed to immense changes in her day-to day mood and general life satisfaction.

In summary, she had gone from a person living in a homeless shelter for battered women, cutting herself every day, battling regular suicidality, to a young lady who had decreased her cutting by 400 %, had a part-time job, was splitting apartment rent with a roommate, and was dating an apparently relatively healthy man who, over two months of dating, had demonstrated no huge "red flags."

I have been more wordy in setting up this tool than most; however, I believe this is an important area to address. If she had believed her father's statement that she was "not getting any better," this would have been incredibly disheartening. The reality is that she had not stopped her cutting completely yet (which was her goal); but it was wonderful for her that she had an entire list of evidence that she was getting better with which to combat the message she kept hearing from him.

Ways I Know I Am Better

1. _____
2. _____
3. _____
4. _____
5. _____
6. _____
7. _____
8. _____
9. _____
10. _____

Tool #13: Distress Tolerance

Sensations

Many people with BPD find that sensations can often help modulate intense emotions. Use the following tool to help you evaluate methods of using the five senses to assist in regulating your emotions. Examples from clients are listed, but as always feel free to come up with your own in each category as well.

- **Hearing:** The following sounds (i.e., music, relaxation CDs, running water, birds chirping, etc.) can be soothing to me _____

_____

_____

- **Sight:** The following things I can see (i.e., paintings, other artwork, calming scenes, clouds, other sights in nature, etc.) can be soothing to me _____
_____
_____

- **Smell:** The following smells (i.e., incense, candles, aromatherapy, pine trees, fabric softener, etc.) can be soothing for me _____
_____
_____

- **Taste:** The following tastes (i.e., chocolate, raisins, ice cream, chewing gum, candy or lasagna) can be soothing to me _____
_____
_____

- **Touch:** The following things I can touch (i.e., stuffed animals, comfy PJs, freshly washed sheets, massage, etc.) can be soothing to me _____
_____
_____

Soothing Strategies

Many individuals with BPD were not soothed as children. Some were severely abused or neglected, and others were simply parented by mothers who were not overly nurturing. Also, some people are born with a predisposition to be more sensitive than others. When needs are not met or feelings get hurt, it is important to have a set of coping skills that can help de-escalate our emotions. If you have a friend who has a calming effect on you, connecting with that person is often a preferable way to alleviate intense emotions. However, people are often not available when we need them. So it is also important to have some ways to self-soothe. A soothing strategy might be defined as *any coping skill that has a calming effect or helps one to relax in some way.* The tools related to connecting to the senses referenced above fit in this category. Other commonly-used soothing strategies include taking a bubble bath, getting a massage, listening to calming music, applying lotion, watching a sunset, enjoying nature, and snuggling with a pet. Use the following tool to identify skills that you might use in this area.

- **Soothing strategies I might use** _____

_____
_____
_____
_____
_____
_____
_____

Distraction Techniques

A distraction technique might be defined as *any coping skill that requires thought*. For instance, taking a hot bath may be a good coping skill, but does it inherently require thought? A question to ask is: Can I still do this behavior and continuously stew on my upsetting thoughts? In the case of a bath: Yes, it is possible to stare at the tiles in front of you and obsess over whatever has you worked up. So technically, a bath would not fit this definition of distraction. On the other hand, writing a letter to someone requires you to think about what you are writing. Since we can't think two thoughts at the same time, letter writing offers periods when we are focused off of the upsetting topic. Sometimes, you may experience intrusive thoughts "jumping back" in your mind, but if that is the case, you can get at least temporary relief. And it is also possible that the topic of your distraction will "take over" for a while and you may not think of the distressing event again for some period of time. It should be noted that distraction can be unhealthy if it feeds your avoiding an event or topic you need to confront. Distraction techniques are only healthy when used as *temporary* measures to decrease the intensity of your mood, so that you can be calmer and in a more rational place to confront events that need to be dealt with and to process them so they no longer affect you negatively. Use this tool to list some distraction techniques that come to mind that you might try.

1. _____

2. _____

3. _____

4. _____

5. _____

Tool #14: Developing Your Identity

Finding identity is a lifetime struggle for some with BPD. It is not an exercise you can do once or twice and be done; it requires ongoing and intentional work. Use the following tool to help you devise a strategy to develop identity.

One of the diagnostic criteria of BPD is "identity disturbance." Many people wrestle with the issue of identity in different ways. While this may look or feel different in different people, persons with BPD often say variations of "I just don't know who I am." This may look different in terms of behaviors. Difficulty establishing hobbies, indecision when choosing a college major, having confusion in relation to sexual or occupational preference, frequently shifting values can all be manifestations of this criteria. It is also common for people with BPD to be so consumed with being who others what them to be and deferring to what others what them to do, that they never really develop a true identity of their own.

While developing identity is certainly not attainable in a certain session or with a single tool, searching for anchors around which to develop healthy self identity can be a worthwhile endeavor.

Finding identity starts with answering the question, *"how do I define myself?"*

You have probably heard the expression that someone "wears a lot of hats." This refers to the various roles the person plays in life. Some people assign more meaning to those roles than others. Thus, they become more important part parts of their identity.

People define themselves by virtue of their relationships to other people, affiliations to religious groups, hobbies, occupations, or a particular areas of interest they have, just to name a few. For instance, one client's included being a niece, a sister, a friend, a Christian, a church member, a stamp collector, a taxi cab driver, a secretary, and a moviegoer.

Use the following tool to identify some of the hats that you wear. Write these in under various hats in the illustration. These roles that you play in life can then be used to work on developing a healthy sense of self identity.

The Hats Tool

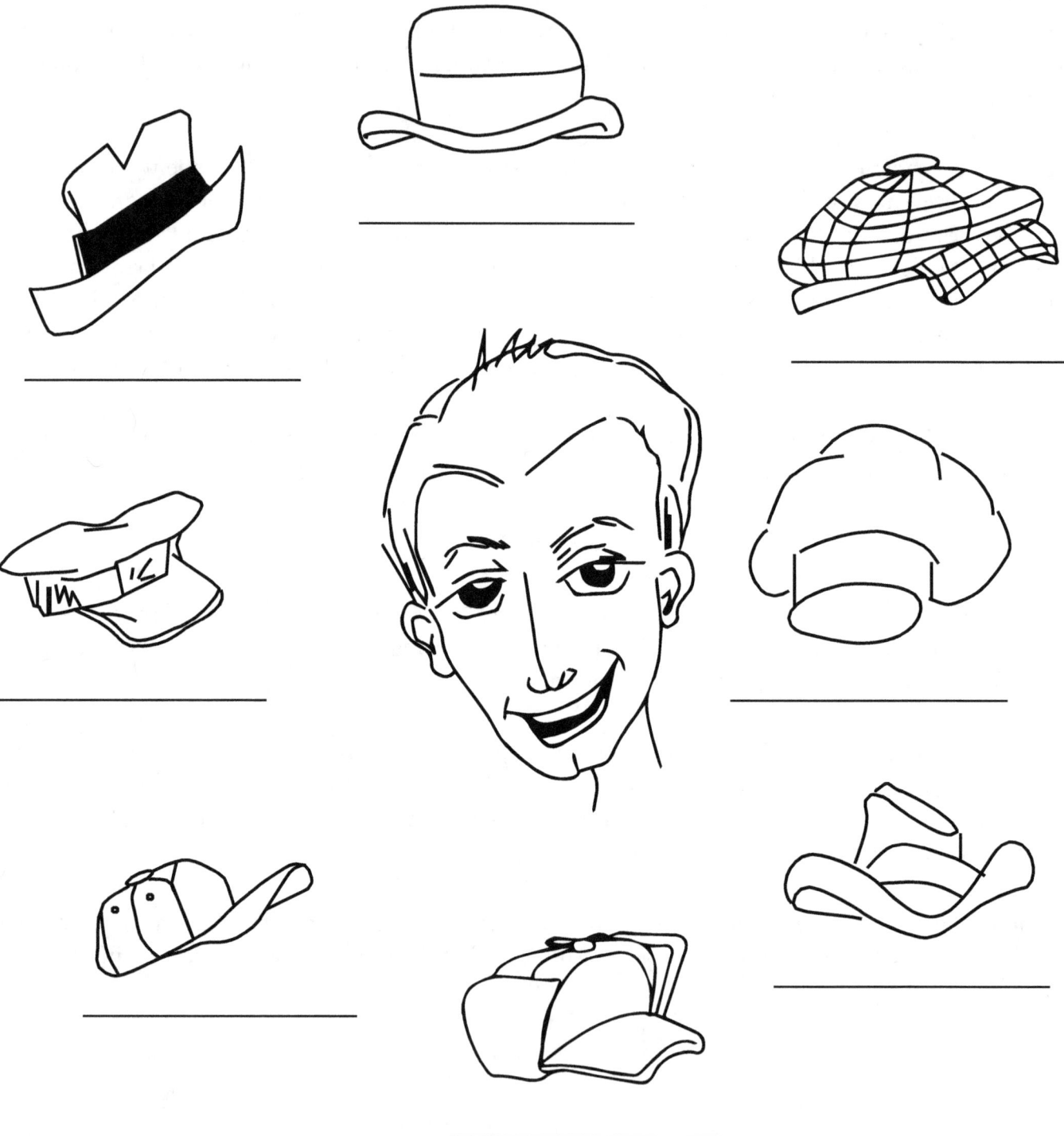

Adapted from Velasquez, Maurer, Crouch, and DiClemente, 2001

- The hat I identify with most _____

Page 288 The Personality Disorders Toolbox: The Challenge of the Hidden Agenda

- The hat I identify with least _____

- Three ways I can expand my identity as a _____ are
  (hat that means the most to me)

  1. _____
  2. _____
  3. _____

Tool #15: Self-Therapy Session—Schema Modification Work

This final tool offers a little bit deeper work that often requires the assistance of a therapist for maximum benefit. But let me give you a sneak peak into what would happen in a therapy session for somebody with BPD doing schema modification work. Note that this is not all of what schema therapy does; in fact, it is hardly even the tip of the iceberg. But modification of those underlying structures that drive thoughts, feelings, and behaviors is more difficult with individuals with PDs and is vital for sustained growth. Also note that this deeper work is only done after life interfering behaviors no longer persist.

First, a little more socialization to the schema model. In his self-help book *Reinventing Your Life,* Jeff Young details what working with this model might look like from a lay perspective. He describes how there are three different coping styles that can make the same schema manifest in different ways. That is why you could have three people with BPD walk through your office door on the same day and they could all three present completely differently. The coping styles are what he calls maintenance ("surrender"), *avoidance,* and *overcompensation* ("counterattack").

So, for instance, the belief (schema) that says, "I can't be okay alone," could manifest different behaviors in different people:

1. Maintenance – This is where one gives in to the belief and follows through with the behavior. In my training sessions, I often share with my clients the visual of an arm-wrestling match: When you are arm wrestling someone a bit stronger than you, you eventually, slowly, give in. Similarly, with the surrender style, one gives in to the belief and engages in the behavior. Some examples of surrender behaviors that could be produced from the example belief of "not being okay alone" include smothering behaviors, constant phone calls, staying in an abusive relationship for an extended period of time, "settling" for the first option that comes along the minute one relationship ends, and so on.

2. Avoidance – This is where one avoids situations that would trigger the belief. Avoidant behaviors produced by this belief might include surface level conversation, not opening up, only sharing superficial details about self, limiting time spent with someone, or any other behavior enacted with the goal of avoiding emotional attachment.

3. Overcompensation – This is where one acts exactly *opposite* of the belief in an extreme way. Small steps to intentionally confront a maladaptive schema are adaptive. DBT uses a term called "opposite action" that often applies to this. But overcompensation is (often unconsciously) acting drastically opposite of a schema, thereby reinforcing it. Some example manifestations of the example belief might include quitting a job before getting fired, dumping a partner before being broken up with, or any number of other types of sabotaging behaviors.

The first step is to do/receive the psychoeducation to make sure the person doing the work understands their style. As awareness increases, clients (at first, in session) should be able to:

1. Identify target behaviors that they observed in the previous week,

2. Identify the belief that the behaviors were a product of,

3. Identify the category of coping style, and

4. List 3 alternative behaviors they could have done instead in the moment

Session agendas will typically include a mood check, a review of homework from the previous session, and then walk through the process described above. Responses are processed with the professional and or group members. Once clients demonstrate the ability to do this with the assistants of a therapist, the frequency of individual sessions can than be decreased. At this point it can be helpful to have clients do their own "self-therapy" sessions at home during off weeks that they don't have appointments. This can reinforce new learning and help facilitate mastery. Clients can use the following tool as a guideline for these "self-therapy appointments."

Self-Therapy Session Tool

Date _____   Session # _____

❏ Depression   ❏ Anxiety   ❏ Anger

Safety Issues Y/N   If so, refer to your safety plan or call your therapist.

If no, great! Move on to behavioral pattern breaking agenda.

- One behavior I enacted this week that was a product of the belief I am targeting
  _____

- This was a product of my _____ belief.

- It was in the (circle one) Maintenance/ Avoidance /Overcompensation category.

- Three things I could have done instead in that moment which would not have reinforced my unhealthy belief and which would have reinforced my heathy belief

    1. _____
    2. _____
    3. _____

Today's Learning Point _____

_____
_____
_____
_____
_____

CHAPTER 10:
THE SCHIZOID AND SCHIZOTYPAL PERSONALITY DISORDER

The Schizoid and Schizotypal Personality Disorder

The schizoid and the schizotypal personality disorders will be combined into one chapter because, frankly, there isn't as much to say about them. It is believed that these disorders share neurological, psychophysiological, and behavioral characteristics associated with disorders of the schizophrenia spectrum. Many of you probably noticed that DSM 5 went ahead and listed schizotypal PD with the schizophrenia spectrum disorders. It did not list schizoid PD there at this point, however.

Practically speaking, we know that we see very few of these folks in the clinical setting. They are among the least interested in treatment, and they probably are the least responsive to psychotherapeutic intervention.

Having said that, this chapter will be an abbreviated one. It will still provide basic demographic information, cognitive profiles, and behavioral targets for each. It will offer an explanation of how each of the tools effective across disorders (Tools #1-9 in each chapter) might be used with each of the two, but will not give detailed examples. Refer to Chapters 1 through 8 for examples. A few schizoid and schizotypal-specific tools will then be offered.

The Schizoid Personality Disorder

Hidden agenda: To not be bothered

Prevalence rates: Approximately 1% of the general population

Gender distribution: More commonly diagnosed in men than women

Cognitive profile:

- View of self: "I am enough"

- View of others: "Others are unnecessary"

- View of world: "The world is boring"

Common schemas: Emotional inhibition, emotional deprivation, negativity

Common cognitive distortions: Discounting the positive

Overdeveloped traits: Autonomy, isolation

Underdeveloped traits: Intimacy, reciprocity

Whom they date/marry: Nobody

Where they work: Solitary jobs that require intellect but little human contact: shift work, truck drivers, air traffic control, engineers

Other Random Nuggets: More commonly diagnosed in first-degree relatives of individuals with schizophrenia, least hospitalized of any personality disorder

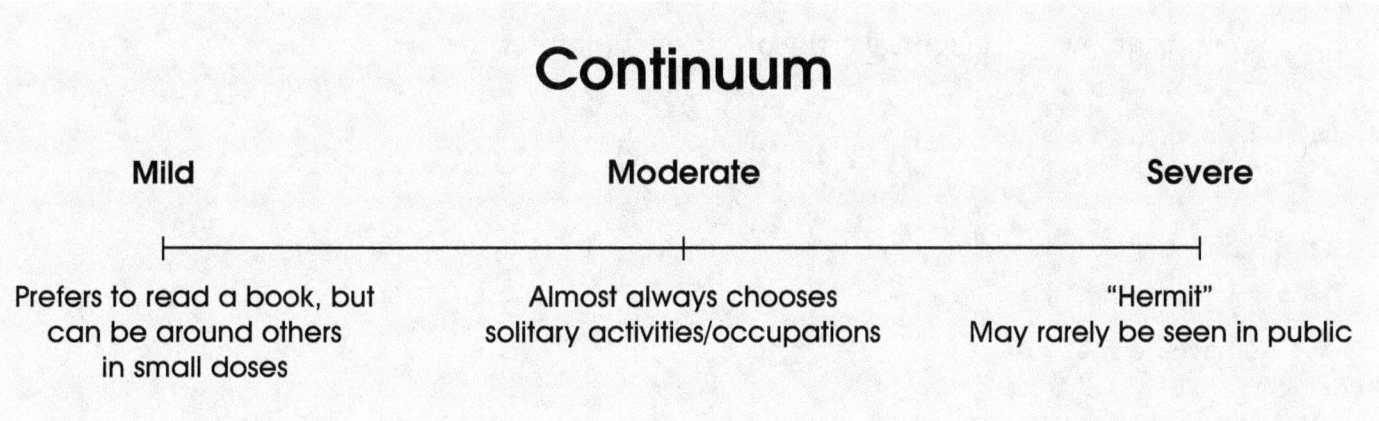

Schizoid personality disorder (SPD) is basically characterized by avoiding people and being fine with it. People with avoidant personality disorder, as well as basic social anxiety or shyness, avoid other people as well, but they have anxiety about it because, deep down, they are people who want relationships but are too scared of being rejected.

People with schizoid traits don't *want* relationships. One of the diagnostic criteria says: *neither desires nor enjoys close relationships.* In fact, closeness and intimacy is about the only thing that triggers anxiety in this population. They are very detached individuals. Beck said they are "observers of rather than participants in the world around them." (Beck, et. Al, 2006)

If you have SPD, it is unlikely that you are reading this, because people with schizoid traits have very little interest in being different. Also, people with schizoid traits are affectively constricted. That is, they often have a very "flat" or "absent" expression on their face. One family member of a client made the statement about the person: "It's just kind of like he's a failure-to-thrive adult." They can often give that appearance. Also because of this detached, flattened affect and expressionless face, clinicians may believe such individuals are depressed, and they may get misdiagnosed. Although, it can appear as though depression might be the problem; depressed people will tell you how miserable they are. Schizoids will say, "I'm fine." And they mean it. They are in no significant distress. If an SPD individual could find a job that involved no people, they would be in heaven. If others didn't ask them to interact, they'd be perfectly happy. If given a choice to go to a party with friends or read a book at home… well, you get where this is going.

Having summarized the characteristics of this disorder, let's hit the "top of the waves" as far as intervention goes. Expressions of concern are often voiced by spouses (if married, which is less likely in this population) or family members, and typically center around their lack of meeting emotional needs. Motivating factors may be more related to space or work concerns, though some will marry and consider to some degree the concerns of a spouse.

Pros and cons as well as target behaviors typically center around isolation. Relationship circles are often nearly completely empty. Schema, thought log, and evidence work usually focuses on tolerating closeness to the degree that is necessary in order to function successfully in society.

Some common automatic thoughts worthy of consideration for therapy include:

- "I'd rather be alone"

- "I'd rather do it myself"

- "I have no motivation"

- "You might as well just go through the motions"

Research is slim when it comes to SPD, but it is believed that emotional neglect may serve as a significant environmental risk factor combining with what is likely a heavily loaded genetic predisposition to produce this condition.

"Why Bother" Tool

If you have SPD, this very well may be your motto. And this is a good question. If your actions are not hurting yourself or anyone else, you may be correct that there is no reason for you to mess around in the lives of other people. If it begins causing problems for you or those who affect you in some way, then you have some decisions to make. The following tool asks you to think about when it is in your best interest to "bother" and when it is not.

Areas of My Life I Can Keep to Myself	Areas of My Life Which Keeping to Myself Causes Problems

Schizoid Task Tool

While neuroscience now tells us that the whole "left brain-right brain" thing is a bit of a misnomer, as the brain is not as dichotomous as we once believed, many therapists and coaches continue to use this outdated language. Having said that, people with schizoid traits would fall on the far end of the spectrum that used to be called "left brain." They are the epitome of the rational, analytical "thinker" that is diametrically opposed to the "right brain" "feeler."

People with schizoid traits can harness this idea when selecting strategies for getting better. For instance, I once had a schizoid patient get involved in a local math club. It was a way for him to feed his desire for intellectual pursuits, while doing so with a only few people with whom he had something in common. These people were almost as uncomfortable with intimacy as he was, so conversations remained pretty comfortable for him. And he eventually made the best two friends he ever had in his life.

Use the following tool to identify some activities that fit in this domain. Put an "X" by the ones you may be willing to try. Feel free to add your own. See if you can identify an area you would be willing to pursue and allow your therapist to probe you to become a little more active in your desired niche.

- ❏ Browse the Apple store
- ❏ Buy new electronic gadgets
- ❏ Teach a class
- ❏ Collect something of interest
- ❏ Follow a blog of interest
- ❏ Plan daily schedules
- ❏ Attend conferences in niche area
- ❏ Generate daily "to do" lists
- ❏ Learn online marketing
- ❏ Take up photography
- ❏ Get a magazine or online subscription
- ❏ Get involved (responsibly) in the stock market
- ❏ Start a You Tube channel teaching people your craft
- ❏ _____
- ❏ _____
- ❏ _____
- ❏ _____
- ❏ _____

- One step I am willing to take to pursue an area of interest _____
_____
_____

Pleasurable Events Tool

Although beginning with the traditional "left-brain" types of tasks is often a helpful starting point, introducing more "right-brain" activities over time can really help individuals with schizoid traits break through the detachment and connect more with their feelings. Experiencing positive emotions can be a new, scary, and extremely powerful phenomenon for people with these characteristics. Consider the following list of ideas that could help you experience positive emotions, and put an "X" by the one's you may be willing to try.

- ❑ Listen to music
- ❑ Lay in the sun
- ❑ Take a hot bath
- ❑ Collect something of interest
- ❑ Go to the pool/beach
- ❑ Kissing
- ❑ Watch a move
- ❑ Go to a picnic
- ❑ Take a road trip or vacation
- ❑ Go see a comedian

- ❑ Work on car or other project
- ❑ Exercise
- ❑ Start a You Tube channel teaching people your craft
- ❑ Shoot pool
- ❑ _____
- ❑ _____
- ❑ _____
- ❑ _____
- ❑ _____

- One step I'm willing to take to pursue one of these areas _____

_____

_____

Expressing Anger Tool

Anger is an emotion that is difficult for people with SPD to express. Some people grew up in families where anger was associated with fear. Many people have internalized ideas like, "anger is always bad," or "anger always leads to violence." For others, anger is the only emotion they know—or at least, the only emotion that is acceptable to express. It is common for people who grew up in families where sharing emotions was a sign of weakness to not express them in adulthood. For these individuals, expressing emotions is a sign of vulnerability, which they aren't willing to reveal. Some just would rather avoid the conflict. This likely is the case for most individuals with SPD. Any human interaction is uncomfortable, so conflict must be doubly unpleasant. Anger does not have to be some intense, scary thing. It takes many forms and can be felt or experienced to varying degrees. The reality is that people are not just angry or they aren't. Anger is experienced on a continuum. Annoyed, irritated, frustrated, agitated, mad, upset, perturbed, and enraged are among emotions in the anger feelings family. It is easier for some people to admit, for instance, they are irritated than that they are "angry," because of the association they have with the word. But the reality is that it is a milder version of the same thing.

Holding onto anger at any level is usually bothersome to anyone, though. And since most people with schizoid traits don't care if others are upset, it is usually in their best interest to acknowledge it. Likely the relief you will get from the annoyance will outweigh the discomfort of the interaction.

Use the following tool to identify feelings of anger you have experienced, and consider whom in your life it may be beneficial to express these emotions to.

My anger feelings are

1. _____

2. _____

3. _____

- The person in my life who annoys me the most frequently _____
_____
_____

- When I don't express my irritation _____
_____
_____

- It could benefit me to express my feelings of anger because _____
_____
_____

Tolerating Closeness Tool

Whether you are employed, or part of a family or any other group of people, some level of closeness may be required. If it is a requirement for your life, unless you want to be uncomfortable until you die, you might as well learn to tolerate it. Some with SPD even come to enjoy some level of closeness.

Review the following tips for tolerating closeness and consider what you might be willing to try.

- Identify one or two people with whom you are most comfortable

- Don't change your interactions with anyone else at the beginning

- Start small

- Share superficial details for a period of time before getting personal

- Inform the person(s) of your need to start small

- Ask them to start small so you don't feel overwhelmed

- Examine your thoughts regarding how closeness causing causes uncomfortableness

- Practice, practice, practice

- Be aware ahead of time that you will not like the interaction to begin with

- Be willing to persist, knowing your comfort level will increase over time

- When you want to quit, remind yourself of the benefit and why you are really doing it

My Response _____

_____

_____

The Schizotypal Personality Disorder

Hidden agenda: To discover something exciting

Prevalence rates: 1-5% of the general population

Gender distribution: More commonly diagnosed in men than women

Cognitive profile:

- View of self: "I am unique"

- View of others: "Others are ordinary"

- View of world: "The world is my lab"

Common schemas: Social isolation

Common cognitive distortions: ?

Overdeveloped traits: Curiosity

Underdeveloped traits: Conformity

Whom they date/marry: May not marry, may pick partner with one similar interest (occupational, religious, hobby, etc.)

Where they work: Inventors, palm readers, artists

Other Random Nuggets: Schizotypal personality has been considered an endophenotype for schizophrenia and as such, DSM 5 has officially listed it with the schizophrenia spectrum disorders

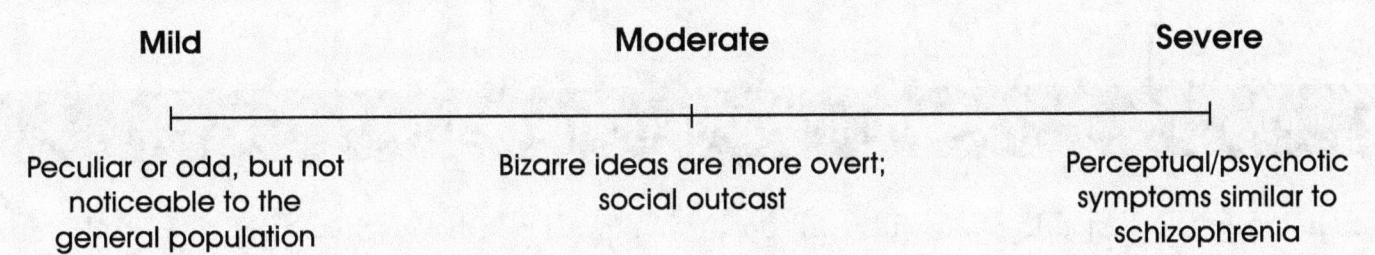

Individuals with schizotypal personality disorder (STPD) have a rich fantasy life and are often more willing to share their odd or even bizarre thoughts than other groups of people. They exhibit social isolation, constricted or situationally inappropriate affect, and unusual behavior. The bizarre thoughts include, but are not limited to, paranoid thinking related to their environment, ideas of reference, and illusions. The odd behaviors are a product of the bizarre thinking, and in fact, cognitive distortions in people with this disorder are perhaps the most severe of any of the personality disorders.

Pros and cons as well as target behaviors typically center around engaging in behaviors that are socially or situationally inappropriate. People with schizotypal traits have people in their circles (see Tool #5 in Chapters 1-8); however, the relationships typically lack depth. Schema, thought log, and evidence work is usually based around the oddities in cognition that produce the inappropriate behaviors.

Some common types of automatic thoughts worthy of consideration in therapy include:

- "He knows what I am thinking"

- "Someone on the TV is watching me"

- "My invention will change the world"

- "The city is doing road work outside my house—they are up to something"

- "Because I am having this thought, it has to be true"

Research is slim when it comes to STPD, but it is believed emotional neglect may play a role, but again, this condition is believed to be highly genetic.

Since the majority of evidence gathered from the research we do have supports three symptom clusters—1) the distorted thinking alluded to above; 2) social deficits; and 3) disorganized behavior)—the tools for this PD will focus on those areas.

Situation Management Tool

This is often the first thing you will work on in therapy. If you have schizotypal traits and are in treatment, you likely have engaged in some type of unusual or inappropriate behavior that has created a situation. Initially, tell your therapist about the situation you are in, and make an attempt, even if it will be difficult, to be open to their feedback.

- Describe the situation _____
  _____
  _____
  _____

- List previous attempts you have made to deal with the situation _____
  _____
  _____

- Suggestions received include
    1. _____
    2. _____
    3. _____

- Something new I am willing to try to manage the situation with _____
  _____
  _____

Medication Compliance Tool

In general, you don't medicate a personality. However, as has been suggested previously, schizotypal disorder is perhaps best not characterized as a personality disorder, but rather as a disorder of psychosis that has interpersonal manifestations.

Since psychotic symptoms often respond to psychotropic medication, pharmacological intervention is often helpful with this population. If this is you, you may want to consider a pro's and cons list of taking medication. Consider and write down all the benefits and drawbacks of taking medications that you can think of, and share them with your therapist.

- Potential benefits of taking medications _____
_____
_____

- Potential drawbacks of taking medications _____
_____
_____

- I am willing to do a trial of a medication recommended for me until the following date _____

Social Skills Training Tool

Increasing social appropriateness can be an invaluable tool for people with STPD. Again, if you have these traits, this probably doesn't sound like your idea of fun. But consider it a social science experiment – see what you can learn! Your therapist may have a local skills training course to refer you to. You could also enlist a friend to take you to one of their social events. Observe and take notes; see what you can learn about socially appropriate behavior.

One of my clients was going to church with a friend of his and afterwards out to lunch with his group of friends. The second time he did this, his friend came back with a story. Apparently, somehow, the group conversation wandered onto the topic of dreams. People were sharing some of their common dreams. To the amazement of my client, several people had experienced the same dreams that he had. So he decided to volunteer one of his dreams. He shared: *"Has anyone had the one where you are living with a warlock and then a girl tries to attack you and you start stabbing her over and over and over until you see blood start running out her of eyes and you realize it is the leader of hell's angels attempting to recruit you?"*

I'll give you one guess as to how this dream went over at the table. I was able to work with my client once I got some ideas from his friend, who accompanied him to therapy, about the kinds of things he was doing and saying. We were than able to do more specific social skills training around some of the things he said in certain social situations.

Take a class recommended by your therapist, plan a social outing with a friend, or engage in any other kind of activity that could expose you to situations that you could observe and/or learn social skills.

- **Social behaviors I have enacted in the past that were considered inappropriate**
  _____
  _____
  _____

- **Takeaways from my social skills class, outing, or activity** _____
  _____
  _____

Jury Duty Tool

If you have ever had jury duty, you know the objective (after you sit in the large room feeling like you are part of a cattle call, waiting to see if you will be selected) is to sit and listen to both sides present their evidence. There are often cases where evidence is collected that suggests the defendant might be innocent, but by the end of trial more evidence comes in that proves he is guilty. The job of the juror is to examine all the evidence fairly; not to let bias enter into the equation or to go by your "gut feeling," but rather to weigh the objective evidence evenly in order to come to conclusions.

For people with STPD, ideas "feel" true that seem bizarre to everyone else. Sometimes it is hard to refute that "gut" feeling. Trusting our "gut" can get any of us in trouble, but it is obviously especially true for people that have more outlandish thoughts and beliefs than they have the insight to be aware of.

Thus, learning how to objectively evaluate evidence for a thought or belief—requiring evidence rather than relying emotional reasoning or "gut" instincts—can be a powerful tool for you if you have these STPD traits. Use the following tool to examine the evidence for some of the thoughts or beliefs your therapist helps you identify.

Idea in Question	Evidence for Idea	Evidence Against Idea

My Final Verdict (for now) _____

_____

_____

Putting Away The Crystal Ball Tool

One specific type of distorted thinking seen in many clients with STPD is what is called *magical thinking*. This occurs when a person mistakenly misinterprets the relationship between given actions and life events.

I had a client who heard a story on the news that particular day that mentioned trouble in the Middle East. When he came to my office that day, he said, "I was thinking about the Middle East today, so that means the news anchors know what I'm thinking." After looking at a number of alternative explanations, he was able to come to the conclusion, "I guess I don't have a crystal ball."

The following tool provides a format for you to identify your "magical thinking" and consider some alternative explanations. It will then ask to you rate the believability of your reasoning on a scale of 0-10, indicating the extent to which you believe your belief versus the alternatives.

Magical Thinking	Alternative Explanations	Rating

My "Reality Testing" Conclusions _____
_____
_____

Goal Setting Tool

The final tool here is a simple one. It simply involves asking yourself, "What are my goals?" Sometimes people try to change us in ways that are not necessary. It is possible to behave in ways that are peculiar to others and to still achieve our goals at the same time. As long as behaviors are not causing problems in important areas of life, be yourself! Use this tool to identify goals you can achieve without hurting yourself or others while remaining "eccentric."

My Goals

1. _____

2. _____

3. _____

- Odd thinking and behavior I recognize in myself which I should be aware of

_____

_____

_____

CONCLUSION

Conclusion

In conclusion, I am happy that I wrote this book. It may not be a best-seller like my first two books, or win an award like my first second book. I get that. I even had people urge me not to write the book because "trying to target ALL personality disorders is too broad," and "too few people have some of the disorders so it will be a waste of time."

I happen to believe that if even a few people benefit from this book it is worth it. There has been nothing out there for some people. And now there is. And we know these tools work.

There are a few caveats.

If you are a patient or mental health consumer, it may be necessary to work through these with the assistance of a skilled therapist. It is possible to make a concerted effort to try the tools, but have difficulty implementing them effectively on your own.

If you are a provider, first and foremost, they have to be implemented within the context of a genuine therapeutic relationship with at least some degree of mutual trust. Perhaps this should have been the first thing I addressed in the book. Or perhaps it goes without saying that you have to be a real person who genuinely wants to help other people. If not, they will see right through you. You also have to be relatable and have the ability to meet clients where they are at. Finally, you have to have some therapeutic instinct that guides your decisions with regard to which tools to use with which clients, and gives you a reasonable sense of when to use what. That is, you have to be able to recognize situations that call for something other than a hammer and know how to use the other tools as well.

Whether you are a professional or a consumer, I appreciate your interest in my *Toolbox* series, and I wish you all Godspeed.

. . .

Note: If you are someone or know someone that has Borderline PD that is not able to access treatment, for an educational alternative (or a supplement) contact me at bpdcoach@jeffriggenbach.com.

BIBLIOGRAPHY

Bibliography

Ameli, R. (2014). American Psychological Association. *25 Lessons in Mindfulness: Now Time for Healthy Living*.

Amarine, MC, Frankenburg, FR, Hensen, J, Reich, DB, and Silk, KR. "Predictions of the 10-year course of borderline personality disorder." *American Journal of Psychiatry*, 163:827-832, 2006.

American Psychiatric Association. (2013). *Diagnostic and Statistical Manual of Mental Disorders*. 5th ed. Washington, D.C.: American Psychiatric Association.

American Psychiatric Association. (2007). *Diagnostic and statistical manual of mental disorders, 4th ed, text revision*. Washington, DC: American Psychiatric Association.

American Psychiatric Association. "Practice Guidelines for the Treatment of Patients with Borderline Personality Disorder." *American Journal of Psychiatry*, 158: 1-52, October 2001.

Andrews, D. A., & Botna, J. (2010). *The Psychology of Criminal Conduct* 4th ed. New Providence, NJ: Matthew Bard & Company.

Antony, m. (2008). *The Anti-Anxiety Workbook: Proven Strategies to Overcome Worry, Phobia, Panic, & Obsessions*. Guilford, New York.

Antony, M. (2009). *When Perfect Isn't Good Enough*. New Harbinger, New York.

Appelbaum A. *Supportive Psychotherapy in Textbook of Personality Disorders* (2005), edited by J Oldham, et al. Am Psychiatric Publishing, Inc: Washington DC. 335-346.

Aguirre, B. A. (2007). *Borderline Personality Disorder in Adolescents: A Complete Guide to Understanding and Coping When Your Adolescent Has BPD*. Fair Winds Press.

Lotte L.M. Bamelis, Fritz Renner, David Heidkamp, and Arnoud Arntz (2011). *Extended Schema Mode Conceptualizations for Specific Personality Disorders: An Empirical Study. Journal of Personality Disorders: Vol. 25, No. 1*, pp. 41-58.

Bateman AW, Fonagy P. "Effectiveness of Partial Hospitalization in the Treatment of Borderline Personality Disorder: A Randomized Controlled Trial." *American Journal of Psychiatry.* 156:1563-1569, 1999.

Bateman, A. & Fonagy, P. (2006). *Mentalization Based Therapy for Borderline Personality Disorder: A Practical Guide.* Oxford University Press. Oxford.

Bateman A, Fonagy P. Mentalization-Based Treatment of BPD. *J of Pers Dis* (2004) 18:1; 36-51.

Beck, J. (2011). *Cognitive Therapy for Challenging Problems: What to do when the Basics don't work.* Guildford. New York.

Beck, J. (2011). *Cognitive Behavior Therapy, Second Edition: Basics and Beyond.* Guilford, New York.

Beck, A.T. The Evolution of the Cognitive Model of Depression and its neurobiological correlates. *American Journal of Psychiatry,* 2008.

Beck, A.T. (1999). *Prisoners of Hate: The Cognitive Basis of Anger, Hostility, and Hate.* Harper Collins Publishing. New York.

Beck, AT. (2014). *Cognitive Therapy of Personality Disorders, Third Edition.* Guilford. New York.

Behary, W. (2013). *Disarming the Narcissist.* New Harbinger, New York.

Bender D. *Therapeutic Alliance in Textbook of Personality Disorders* (2005), edited by J Oldham, et al. Am Psychiatric Publishing, Inc: Washington DC. 405-420. Bohus, M., Dyer, A., et al. (2013). *Dialectical Behavior Therapy for Post Traumatic Stress Disorder after childhood sexual abuse in patients with and without borderline personality disorder: a randomized controlled trial.* Psychotherapy and Psychosomatics. 82, 221-223.

Brodsky B. & Stanley, B. (2013). *The Dialectical Behavior Therapy Primer: How DBT can inform clinical practice.* Wiley and Sons, Ltd.

Clark L. Stability and Change in Personality Pathology: Revelations of Three Longitudinal Studies. *J Pers Dis* (2005) 19(5) 524-532.

Clarkin J. et al. Evaluating Three Treatments for Borderline Personality Disorder: A Multiwave Study. *Am J Psych* (June 2007) 164:922-92.

Cloninger CR (edit.) *Personality and Psychopathology.* American Psychiatric Press. Washington, D.C. 1999.

Coccaro E, Siever L. *Neurobiology. in Textbook of Personality Disorders* (2005), edited by J Oldham, et al. Am Psychiatric Publishing, Inc: Washington DC. 155-169.

Cohen P. Child Development and Personality Disorder. *Psych Clin N Am* (2008) 31:477- 493.

Costa P, et al. The Five-Factor Model of Personality and Its Relevance to Personality Disorders. *J Pers Dis* (1992) 6:343-359.

Davidson, Kate. (2000) *Cognitive Therapy for Personality Disorders: A Guide for Clinicians.* Routledge. London.

Farrell, J & Shaw, I. (2012). *Group Schema Therapy for Borderline Personality Disorder: A Step by Step Treatment Manual with Patient Workbook.* Wiley & Sons. West Sussex.

Farrell, JM. (2012). *"Group Schema Therapy".* Encyclopedia of the Science of Learning, 1395-1397.

Freeman, A. & Fusco, G. (1993). *Borderline Personality Disorder: A Patient's Guide to Taking Control.* WW Norton, New York.

Freeman A. Cognitive-Behavior Therapy With Borderline Personality Disorder. *Psychiatric Annals* (June 2004) 34:6; 458-468.

Freeman, Arthur & Fusco, Gina.(2004). *Borderline Personality Disorder: A Therapist's Guide To Taking Control.* W.W. Norton. New York/London.

Friedel, Robert, O. (2004). *Borderline Personality Disorder Demystified.* DaCapo Press. Cambridge.

Gabbard G. Treatment Resistant Borderline Personality Disorder. *Psychiatric Annals* (Nov 1998) 28:11; 651-656.

Gabbard G. *Psychoanalysis. in Textbook of Personality Disorders* (2005), edited by J Oldham, et al. Am Psychiatric Publishing, Inc: Washington DC. 257-273.

Gates, A. & Baker, C. (1995). *The Road to Recovery.* New Forms Press. Stillwater.

Grant B et al. Prevalence, Correlates, Disability, and Comorbidity of DSM-IV Borderline Personality Disorder: Results From the Wave 2 National Epidemiologic Survey on Alcohol and Related Conditions. *J Clin Psych* (April 2008) 69:4;533-545.

Grant, B et al. Prevalence, Correlates, and Disability of Personality Disorders in the United States: Results from the National Epidemiologic Survey on Alcohol and Related Conditions. *J of Clin Psychiatry* (2004) 65;948-958.

Grossman R. Psychopharmacologic Treatment of Patients with Borderline Personality Disorder. *Psychiatric Annals* (June 2002) 32:6 357-370.

Gunderson, JG. (2008). *Borderline Personality Disorder: A Clinical Guide.* American Psychiatric Publishing. Arlington.

Gunderson, J. Borderline Personality Disorder: Ontogeny of a Diagnosis. *Am J Psych* (May 2009) 166:5;530-539.

Gunderson J (2011). Borderline personality disorder. *New England Journal of Medicine*, 364(21): 2037-2042.

Gunderson J, et al. *Levels of Care in Treatment in Textbook of Personality Disorders* (2005), edited by J Oldham, et al. Am Psychiatric Publishing, Inc: Washington DC. 239- 256.

Gunderson, J.G. (2001). *Borderline Personality Disorder: A Clinical Guide.* APA Washington, D.C.

Gunderson J, et al. *Levels of Care in Treatment in Textbook of Personality Disorders* (2005), edited by J Oldham, et al. Am Psychiatric Publishing, Inc: Washington DC. 239- 256.

Hellerstein D, et al. Beyond "Handholding": Supportive Therapy for Patients with BPD and Self-Injurious Behavior. *Psych Times* (July 2004) 58-61.

Hare, R. (1999). *Whithout Conscience.* Guilford, New York.

Herbert, J., & Forman, E. (2011). *Acceptance and Mindfulness in Cognitive Behavior Therapy: Understanding and Applying the New Therapies.* Wiley & Sons. New York.

Jaffee, S., et al. (2006). When Parents Have a History of Conduct Disorder: How is the caregiving environment affected. *Journal of Abnormal Psychology,* Vol 115(2), May, 309-319

Jang K. *The Behavioral Genetics of Psychopathology.* (2005) Lawrence Earlbaum Assoc., Inc, New Jersey.

Jeffries, F.W. & Davis, P. *What is the Role of Eye Movement in EMDR for PTSD? A Review. Behavioral and Cognitive psychotherapy,* 2013, 41, 290-300.

Johnson J, et al. *Role of Childhood Experiences in the Development of Maladaptive and Adaptive Personality Traits, in Textbook of Personality Disorders* (2005), edited by J Oldham, et al. Am Psychiatric Publishing, Inc: Washington DC. 209-221.

Johnson P, et al. Understanding Emotion Regulation in Borderline Personality Disorder: Contributions of Neuroimaging. *Focus* (Summer 2005) 3:3;478-48

Johnson J, et al. *Role of Childhood Experiences in the Development of Maladaptive and Adaptive Personality Traits, in Textbook of Personality Disorders* (2005), edited by J Oldham, et al. Am Psychiatric Publishing, Inc: Washington DC. 209-221.

Johnson P, et al. Understanding Emotion Regulation in Borderline Personality Disorder: Contributions of Neuroimaging. *Focus* (Summer 2005) 3:3;478-483.

Kernberg, Otto, F. (1984). *Severe Personality Disorders.* Yale University Press. New York, London.

Koerner, K. *Doing Dialectical Behavior Therapy.* New York. Guilford.

Kreissman, J. (2006). *Sometimes I Act Crazy.* Wiley, New York.

Kendler KS1, Myers J, Torgersen S, Neale MC, Reichborn-Kjennerud T. *The heritability of cluster A personality disorders assessed by both personal interview and questionnaire.*

Layden, M, Newman, C. (1993) *Cognitive Behavioral Treatment of Borderline Personality Disorder.* Allyn & Bacon, Boston.

Layden, M. A., et al. Cognitive Therapy of Borderline Personality Disorder. Allyn and Bacon. Jang K. *The Behavioral Genetics of Psychopathology.* (2005) Lawrence Earlbaum Assoc., Inc, New Jersey.

Leahy, R. (2011). *Emotion in Psychotherapy.* Guilford, New York.

Leahy, R. (2013). *Cognitive Behavioral Techniques: A Practitioners Guide.* Guilford, New York.

Leahy, R. (2017). *Emotional Schema Therapy.* Guilford, New York.

Lee, C.W & Cuiijpers, Pim. A Meta-analysis of the role of eye movements in processing Emotional Memories. *Journal of Behavioral Therapy and Experimental Psychiatry,* 44, (2013), 231-239.

Lenzenweger M, et al. Individual Growth Curve Analysis Illuminates Stability and Change in Personality Disorder. *Arch of Gen Psychiatry* (Oct 2004) 61; 1015-1024.

Lester, G. (2010). *Personality Disorders in Health Care.* Unpublished.

Lester, G. (1995). *Power with People: How to Handle just about anyone to accomplish just about anything.* Penguine. New York.

Lilienfeld S, et al. The Relationship of Histrionic Personality Disorder to Antisocial Personality and Somatization Disorders. *The Am J of Psychiatry* (June 1986) 143:6; 718- 721.

Linehan M. *Cognitive-Behavioral Treatment of Borderline Personality Disorder.* 1993 New York: Guilford Press.

Linehan, Marsha, et. Al. Reasons for staying alive when you are thinking about killing yourself: The Reasons for Living Inventory. *Journal of Consulting and Clinical Psychology.* 1983, Volume 51, 2, 276-286.

Links P, Kolla N. *Assessing and Managing Suicide Risk in Textbook of Personality Disorders* (2005), edited by J Oldham, et al. Am Psychiatric Publishing, Inc: Washington DC. 449-462.

Lenzenweger M, et al. Individual Growth Curve Analysis Illuminates Stability and Change in Personality Disorder. *Arch of Gen Psychiatry* (Oct 2004) 61; 1015-1024.

Lilienfeld S, et al. The Relationship of Histrionic Personality Disorder to Antisocial Personality and Somatization Disorders. *The Am J of Psychiatry* (June 1986) 143:6; 718- 721.

Lowe J, Widiger T. *Clinicians' Judgments of Clinical Utility: A Comparison of the Dimensional Models of General Personality.* J Pers Dis (2009) 23:3;211-229.

Maddocks P. A Five Year Follow-up of Untreated Psychopaths. *Br J Psych* (1970) 116:511-515.

Malkin, C. (2016). *Rethinking Narcissism.* Harper Perrenial. New York.

Marissa Ericson, Catherine Tuvblad, Adrian Raine, Kelly Young-Wolff, and Laura A. Baker. *Heritability and Longitudinal Stability of Schizotypal Traits During Adolescence.* Behav Genet. 2011 Jul; 41(4): 499–511. Published online 2011 Mar 3. doi: 10.1007/s10519-010-9401

Markovitz P. Recent Trends in the Pharmacotherapy of Personality Disorders. *J of Pers Dis* (2004) 18:1; 90-101.

Marsh A et al. Reduced Amygdala Response to Fearful Expressions in Children and adolescents With Callous-Unemotional Traits and Disruptive Behavior Disorders. *Am J Psych* (June 2008) 165:6;712-720.

Martell, C. R., Dimidjian, S., & Herman-Dunn, R. (2010). *Behavioral Activation for Depression.* Guilford, New York.

Martell D. Neuroscience and the Law: Philosophical Differences and Practical Constraints. *Behav Sci Law* (2009) 27:123-136.

Millon T. *Disorders of Personality.* John Wiley and Sons; New York. 1981.

Morningstar, D. (2017). *Out of the Fog: Moving from Confusin to Clarity After Narcissisti Abuse.*

New A, Siever L. Neurobiology and Genetics of Borderline Personality Disorder. *Psychiatric Annals* (June 2002) 32:6; 329-336.

Novaco, R.W. (2013). Reducing Anger Related Offending: What Works. In L.A. Craig, L. Dixon, & T. A. Gannon (eds.) *What Works in Offender Rehabilitation: An Evidence Based Approach to Assessment and Treatment.* (pp. 211-236). Chicester, UK; John Wiley & Sons, Ltd.

Oldham JM, et al. Practice Guideline for the Treatment of Patients with Borderline Personality Disorder. *Am J of Psychiatry* (2001) 158(10 Suppl):1-52.

Oldham JM. Personality Disorders. *Focus* (Summer 2005) III:8;372-382. Ozarin L. Moral Insanity: A Brief History. *Psych News* (May 2001) 21.

Paris J. Clinical Trials of Treatment for Personality Disorders. *Psych Clin N Am* (2008) 31: 517-526.

Paris, J. (2010). *Treatment of Borderline Personality Disorder: A Guide to Evidence Based Practice.* Guilford, New York.

Paris J. *Personality Disorders Over Time: Precursors, Course, and Outcome.* (2003) Am Psychiatric Publishing, Inc. Arlington, VA.

Paris J. Clinical Trials of Treatment for Personality Disorders. *Psych Clin N Am* (2008) 31: 517-526.

Pederson, L. (2017). *The Expanded Dialectical Behavior Therapy Skills Training Manual.* Pesi Publishing and Media, Eau Claire.

Piper W, et al. *Group Treatment in Textbook of Personality Disorders* (2005), edited by J Oldham, et al. Am Psychiatric Publishing, Inc. Washington DC. 347-357.

Prochaska, J. O., Norcross, J., and DiClemente, C. (2007). *Changing for Good: A Revolutionary six stage program for overcoming bad habits and moving your life positively forward.* Harper Collins. New York.

Riggenbach, J. (2013). *The CBT Toolbox: A Workbook for Clients and Clinicians.* Premiere. Eau Claire.

Riggenbach, J. (2016). *The Borderline Personality Disorder Toolbox: An Evidence-Based Guide for Regulating Emotions.* Pesi Publishing and Media. Eau Claire.

Rizvi S, Linehan M. Dialectical Behavior Therapy for Personality Disorders. *Focus* (Summer 2005) 3:3;489-494. Freeman, A. & Fusco, G. (1993). *Borderline Personality Disorder: A Therapist's Guide to Taking Control.* Norton, New York.

Robinson, D. (2005). *Disordered Personalities.* Rapid Psychler Press. London, Ontario.

Ronningstam E, et al. Changes in Pathological Narcissism. *Am J Psych* (1995) 152:2;253- 257.

Russ E, et al. Refining the Construct of Narcissistic Personality Disorder: Diagnostic Criteria and Subtypes. *Am J Psych* (Nov 2008) 165;11;1473-1481.

Rutter M, et al. Psychosocial Adversities in Psychopathology. *J Pers Dis* (1997) 11:4-18. Sansone R. Chronic Suicidality and Borderline Personality Disorder. *J Pers Dis* (2004) 18:3;215-225.

Schlesinger A, Silk K. *Collaborative Treatment in Textbook of Personality Disorders* (2005), edited by J Oldham, et al. Am Psychiatric Publishing, Inc. Washington DC. 431- 446.

Shea, S.C. (2011). *The Practical Art of Suicide Assessment.* John Wiley. Hoboken, New Jersey.

Silk, K. Borderline Personality Disorder. *Curr Psych* (Nov 2002) 1: 11; 224 -233. Simeon D, et al. Self-Mutilation in Personality Disorders: Psychological and Biological Correlates. *The Am J of Psychiatry* (Feb 1992) 149:2; 221-226. Skeem J, et al. Psychopathy, Treatment Involvement, and Subsequent Violence Among

Skodol A. *Manifestations, Clinical Diagnosis, and Comorbidity in Textbook of Personality Disorders* (2005), edited by J Oldham, et al. Am Psychiatric Publishing, Inc. Washington DC. 57-87.

Soloff P, et al. Self-Mutilation and Suicidal Behavior in Borderline Personality Disorder. *Journal of Pers Dis*, (1994) 8(4); 257-267.

Spear L. The Adolescent Brain and Age-Related Behavioral Manifestations. *Neurosci Biobehav Rev* (2000)24:417-463.

Sperry, Len. (1999). *Cognitive Behavior Therapy of the DSM-IV Personality Disorders.* Brunner-Routledge. New York/London.

Stone M. Perspective: Pitfalls in the Psychotherapy of Borderline Personality or the Triumph of Faith Over Fact. *J Pers Dis* (2009) 23:1;3-5.

Stone M. Personality Disordered Patients: Treatable and Untreatable. 2006. *Am Psychiatric Pub.* Washington, DC.

Stout, M. (2006). *The Sociopath Next Door. Harmony.*

Tafrate, R.(2013) *Forensic CBT: A Handbook for Clinical Practice.* Wiley-Blackwell, New York.

Torgersen S. et al. A Twin Study of Personality Disorders. *Comp Psych* (2000) 41:416- 425.

Turetsky BI1, Calkins ME, Light GA, Olincy A, Radant AD, Swerdlow NR. . Schizophr Bull. 2007 Jan;33(1):69-94. Epub 2006 Nov 29. *Neurophysiological Endophenotypes of Schizophrenia: the Viability of Selected Candidate Measures.*

Torgersen S. "Genetics of Patients with Borderline Personality Disorder." *Psychiatric Clinics of North America.* 23:1-9, 2000.

Verheul R, et al. A Meta-Analysis of the Prevalence and Usage of the Personality Disorder Not Otherwise Specified (PDNOS) Diagnosis. *J Pers Dis* (2004) 18:309-319.

Weber S et al. Structural Brain Abnormalities in Psychopaths: A Review. *Behav Sci Law* (2008) 26: 7-28.

Widiger T. Personality Disorder and Axis I Psychopathology: The Problematic Boundary of Axis I and Axis II. *J of Pers Dis,* (2003) 17(2):90-108.

Yang Y et al. Brain Abnormalities in Antisocial Individuals: Implications for the Law. *Behav Sci Law* (2008) 26:65-83.

Yen S, et al. Traumatic Exposure and Posttraumatic Stress Disorder in Borderline, Schizotypal, Avoidant, and Obsessive-Compulsive Personality Disorders: Findings from the Collaborative Longitudinal Personality Disorders Study. *The J of Nerv and Ment Dis* (2002) Vol. 190, No. 8; 510-518.

Young, J. (2006) *Schema Therapy: A Practitioner's Guide.* Guilford, New York.

Young, J. (1994). *Reinventing Your Life. Plume.* New York.